POSTURE

AND

PAIN

By
HENRY O. KENDALL
Director, Physical Therapy Department

FLORENCE P. KENDALL
Assistant Director, Physical Therapy Department

and

DOROTHY A. BOYNTON
Physical Therapist

Physical Therapy Department
Children's Hospital School
Baltimore, Maryland

fascimile of 1967 edition

ROBERT E. KRIEGER PUBLISHING CO. INC.
Huntington, New York

original edition 1952

reprinted 1955, 1958, 1960, 1963, 1967, 1970, 1975, 1977

printed and published by
Robert E. Krieger Publishing Co. Inc.
Huntington, New York 11743

reprinted by arrangement

ISBN 0-88275-031-3

Printed in U.S.A. by
NOBLE OFFSET PRINTERS, INC.
NEW YORK 3, N. Y.

DEDICATED TO

GEORGE E. BENNETT, M.D.

FOREWORD

In this book on Posture and Pain, Mr. and Mrs. Kendall have set forth the fruit of two lifetimes of experience. To one who has watched them acquire this experience the hard way, it is a very happy task to be asked to write a foreword to their book.

First of all they mastered the technique of accurate muscle testing and evaluation and piled up for later analysis continuing records of individual muscle disturbances, chiefly on poliomyelitis cases. Then came a phase when their interest shifted more to faulty body mechanics and to this problem they brought the same careful analysis of the muscle factors and were stimulated to further clinical research into normal posture. This led to new discoveries as to the normal variations in spine mobility to be expected during the growth period in children. Later they made their excursions to West Point and the Johns Hopkins Nursing School to study and analyze the posture variations in active, normal adults. Finally they went back to the disabled group again and from all their careful records made the final evaluations which this text embodies.

Naturally, the book contains a restatement of many established anatomical and physiological axioms, but it also adds much that is new and eliminates many old false conceptions. Its great value lies in the soundness of their analyses and evaluation and in the clarity with which they have illustrated the text.

The Kendalls have had to have perfect teamwork, rare technical skill, great tenacity of purpose and tireless enthusiasm to accomplish it.

ROBERT W. JOHNSON, *Adjunct Professor*
of Orthopedic Surgery, The Johns Hopkins Medical School

PREFACE

The basic thesis of this book is the importance of postural faults in disabling and painful conditions. The object is to reduce the complexities of postural analysis to the simplest forms, to help solve the problem by presenting the basic therapeutic procedures, and to stimulate an interest in the prevention of postural faults.

This book is intended for those in the medical profession and allied fields who deal with problems of painful conditions resulting from faulty posture. It is also intended for those interested in the development of good posture.

To accomplish its objectives, this book has been extensively illustrated and presented in such a manner that the reader may understand its content without a background of highly specialized training. When technical terms have been used they have been defined at the beginning of the section in which they appear.

This book is divided into four parts. The first is an analysis of good and faulty alignment; the second, an analysis of faults in mobility; the third, the treatment of painful postural conditions; and the fourth, a discussion of some of the developmental factors and environmental influences affecting posture. This presentation brings to anyone dealing with the problem of postural faults findings from a wide experience in testing for and treating such faults.

The physical therapy department at the Children's Hospital School in Baltimore has had over 10,000 admissions between 1932 and 1950. Most of these cases represent some form of orthopedic disability, the majority having been about equally divided between poliomyelitis and faulty or painful postural conditions. Patients with paralytic poliomyelitis often present the extreme in potential or actual faults of alignment and muscle balance. Thus, most of the 10,000 patients have had some associated problem of faulty body mechanics. In addition there have been approximately 2,000 posture examinations of so-called normals in ages ranging from five to twenty-five. With few exceptions, these individuals have been examined by the senior author of this book.

The detailed records of the aforementioned 12,000 cases are on file in the department and, although no tabulation of data is included in this volume, the observations, conclusions, and recommendations presented are based on the experience gained from this large number of cases. This experience has repeatedly demonstrated the relationships which we present, and which we attempt to clarify, illustrate, and interpret for our readers.

In the preparation of the manuscript we sought the advice and guidance of our medical directors, Dr. George E. Bennett and Dr. Robert W. Johnson, Jr. Both are outstanding authorities in the field of orthopedic surgery and we are deeply grateful for their assistance.

Doctors on the staff and others not connected with the hospital have referred cases to the out-patient department. We are grateful to these doctors for these referrals because, as physical therapists, the work of the authors has necessarily been limited to treatment of referred cases. Throughout the years, Dr. Raymond E. Lenhard and Dr. H. Alvan Jones have shown special interest in the problems of faulty body mechanics, and in the referral of such cases.

Dr. Joseph Lilienthal has reviewed Chapter VII, "Pain Associated with Faulty Body Mechanics," and has made valuable suggestions which we have gratefully adopted. The manuscript has been read by Dr. Leonard T. Peterson, and we wish to thank him, also, for his suggestions.

For most of the photographs of adult male subjects shown in this book, we gratefully acknowledge the contribution of the United States Military Academy at West Point. This valuable addition has been made possible through the interest and effort of Colonel F. M. Greene, Director of Physical Education. The postures shown are those of cadets on the day of entrance to the Academy and are the initial record in the splendid posture training program that prevails at West Point.

We wish to acknowledge the cooperation of the faculty and students of the Johns Hopkins Hospital School of Nursing in obtaining most of the photographs of the adult female subjects. We appreciate the skill and care with which these and numerous other photographs were taken by Charles C. Krausse, Jr.

To the Board of Education of Baltimore County, to Mr. Melvin Cole and his staff at Loch Raven Elementary School, and to Mr. Herbert Steiner we extend our sincere thanks for their cooperation in obtaining a series of photographs of children.

Our good friend and able advisor, Mr. Bancroft Hill, was consulted on matters of terms and principles relating to engineering and mechanics. The anatomical drawings have been done by Mr. William Loechel. The authors' desire to capture a specific "feeling" or "attitude" in many of these simple line drawings would not have been realized but for the patience and cooperation of the artist.

We are most grateful for the generous assistance afforded by the Children's Hospital School through the Thomas Henry Bowles Memorial Fund. We also wish to express our thanks to Mrs. Henry Straus and Mr. John McGrath for their generous contributions.

We wish to thank the members of the staff at the Children's Hospital School for their constructive criticism in reviewing the manuscript, for the encouragement they have given us, and for their help in innumerable details. We especially thank Beulah Connaway and Margaret Gold for their help. We also wish to express our sincere appreciation to Ruth P. Stein for her assistance.

We wish to acknowledge the contribution made by the many visitors to the department who have, by their interest and questions, stimulated and clarified our thinking. Their enthusiasm for the interpretation we offered of the basic principles in the fields of body mechanics and poliomyelitis has given us confidence to proceed in our efforts to define and present these principles.

To the publishers, The Williams and Wilkins Company, we extend our most sincere appreciation. We acknowledge also the use of some photographs relating to muscle testing from *Muscles, Testing and Function*, by Henry O. and Florence P. Kendall, The Williams and Wilkins Co., 1949.

CONTENTS

INTRODUCTION

Good posture is a good habit. Once well established it should take little voluntary effort to maintain it. Attainment of good posture should not be regarded as a rigid disciplinary measure, but rather as the development of a habit which contributes to the well-being of the individual.

Conversely, bad posture is a bad habit, unfortunately of relatively high incidence. Despite the prevalence of postural faults in adults it should be recognized that the structure and functions of the human body provide all the potentialities for good posture. The postural faults find their origin, not in the structure of the normal body, but in the mis-use of the capacities provided.

If postural faults were simply an aesthetic problem the concern about them might be limited to concern about appearance. However, it must be recognized that postural faults which persist may cause discomfort, pain, or deformity. The range of effect from discomfort to incapacitating disability is related to the severity of the fault and its persistence.

The motive for this book springs from a recognition of the prevalence of postural faults, the associated pain, and the subsequent waste of human resources. It aims to contribute to a decrease in the incidence of such faults and the resulting pain by defining the concept of good posture, analyzing postural faults, presenting examination and treatment procedures, and discussing some of the developmental factors and environmental influences affecting posture.

In order to achieve the highest degree of well-being, as related to posture, in the cultural pattern of modern civilization, it is essential to recognize the increasing stresses put on the basic structures of the human body by increasingly specialized and limited activity. It is necessary to provide, as far as possible, compensatory influences in order to achieve the optimum result possible under the conditions imposed by our mode of life. The high incidence of postural faults in adults is related to this tendency toward a specialized and consequently a limited or repetitive pattern of activity. Correction of the existing conditions depends on an understanding of the underlying influences, and a program of preventive and positive educational measures. Both of the foregoing rest upon an understanding of the mechanics of the body and its response to the stresses and strains imposed upon it.

An analysis of good and faulty body mechanics in terms of skeletal alignment, joint motion, and muscle action is presented in Chapters I through VI which comprise Parts I and II of this book. Chapter I illustrates and describes an ideal alignment. This alignment, presented by the authors as a standard, is illustrated by detailed line drawings and photographs. Chapter II portrays and analyzes a wide variety of postural faults. The presentation rests upon a series of photographs chosen, from over a thousand pictures, to illustrate the various faults.

Chapter III gives a detailed description of the relationship of the pelvis to the lower extremities and to the spine. This relationship is described and illustrated in detail because the position of the pelvis is regarded as the keynote of postural alignment. Line drawings have been used to illustrate this material.

The importance of muscle testing to posture analysis cannot be over-emphasized. Chapters IV and V describe and illustrate the muscle testing essential to an analysis of posture. Much of the specific therapy in postural correction is based directly on the examination findings in regard to muscle tightness or weakness. Line drawings and photographs have been used to illustrate the test findings. Chapter VI deals with the procedure of an examination, presents photographs of a case, the case record with findings, and the treatment indicated.

Part III deals with the treatment of painful

1

conditions associated with faulty posture. Chapter VII is devoted to a discussion of the mechanism of pain as related to postural faults, and to a presentation of specific treatment modalities. The following two chapters give the analysis of and treatment for various painful conditions. Specifically, Chapter VIII deals with painful conditions of the low back, leg, knee, and foot; Chapter IX, with the upper back, neck, and arm.

Part IV, that is Chapter X, discusses some of the significant factors affecting posture developmentally, and suggests practical approaches for creating a good environment for the development and subsequent naintenance of good postural habits.

PART I

ALIGNMENT

CHAPTER I

THE STANDARD POSTURE

An evaluation of postural faults necessitates a standard by which individual postures can be judged. The alignment used as standard must be consistent with sound scientific principles. It should be the kind of posture which involves a minimal amount of stress and strain and which is conducive to maximal efficiency in the use of the body.* The standard must meet these requirements if the whole system of posture training that is built around it is to be sound.

The *Standard Posture* as used and described in this text refers to an "ideal" posture rather than an average posture. In this chapter the authors illustrate and describe it in specific terms. Its relationship to significant anatomical, physiological, and mechanical factors is discussed in detail. It is important that the reader visualize this standard as a basis for comparison, since good alignment or postural faults will be described in terms of this standard.

The standard is one of *skeletal alignment* because posture is basically a matter of alignment. The body contour in the illustrations of the standard posture is included because it shows the relationship of skeletal structures to surface outline when alignment is excellent. It is recognized that there are variations in body type and size among individuals, and that shape

* A good definition of posture appears in "Posture and its Relationship to Orthopaedic Disabilities," a report of the Posture Committee of the American Academy of Orthopaedic Surgeons, 1947.

"Posture is usually defined as the relative arrangement of the parts of the body. Good posture is that state of muscular and skeletal balance which protects the supporting structures of the body against injury or progressive deformity irrespective of the attitude (erect, lying, squatting, stooping) in which these structures are working or resting. Under such conditions the muscles will function most efficiently and the optimum positions are afforded for the thoracic and abdominal organs. Poor posture is a faulty relationship of the various parts of the body which produce increased strain on the supporting structures and in which there is less efficient balance of the body over its base of support."

and proportions of the body are factors in weight distribution. Nevertheless, the authors believe that a standard of skeletal alignment can be considered a valid standard for evaluating the posture of any individual regardless of body type or size. The importance of body contour lies chiefly in the fact that variations in contour are correlated to some degree with variations in skeletal alignment. Fortunately this is essentially true of every one regardless of bodybuild. Thus an experienced observer is able, by observing the contours of the body, to estimate the position of the skeletal structures.

The standing position may be regarded as the composite alignment of a subject from four views, front, back, right side, and left side. It involves the position and alignment of so many joints and parts of the body that it is not probable that any individual can meet this standard in every respect. As a matter of fact, the authors have not seen an individual who matches the standard in all respects.

The standard posture is illustrated from front, back, and side by line drawings. In the drawings showing the front and back views of the body the vertical *line of reference* represents a plane which coincides with the midline of the body. It is illustrated as beginning midway between the heels and extending upward midway between the lower extremities, through the midline of the pelvis, spine, sternum, and skull. The right and left halves of the skeletal structures are essentially symmetrical and by hypothesis the two halves of the body exactly counterbalance. (See figs. 1, 3 and 5.)

In the side-view drawing the vertical *line of reference* represents a plane which hypothetically divides the body into front and back sections of equal weight. These sections are not symmetrical and there is no obvious line of division on the basis of anatomical structures. It is necessary, therefore, to describe the relationship of the body to this plane on the basis of the mechanical and physiological factors involved. Because this description requires a rather lengthy discussion it appears later in this chapter.

The intersection of these two mid-planes of the body forms a line which is analogous to the gravity line. Around this line the body is hypothetically in a position of equilibrium. This implies a balanced distribution of weight, and a stable position of each joint. Along the course of each line of reference are certain *points of reference*. In the drawings of the standard posture these are shown as deep structures.

The lines and points of reference discussed above are put to practical use in *plumb line tests* for postural alignment. For the purpose of testing, the subject steps up to a suspended plumb line. In back or front view he stands so that the feet are equidistant from the line; in side view, so that the point just in front of the lateral malleolus (in adults about an inch in front of the center of the malleolus) is in line with the plumb line. Thus the *base* points of reference indicated on the drawings of the standard posture are the points in line with which the plumb line is suspended. It is necessary that the base point be the fixed reference point because the base is the only stationary or fixed part of the standing posture.

A plumb line test is used to determine whether the *points of reference* of the individual being tested are in the same alignment as are the corresponding points in the standard posture. The amount of deviation of the various points of reference from the plumb line reveal the extent to which the subject's alignment is faulty. Whenever deviations from plumb alignment are evaluated they are described as slight, moderate, or marked, rather than in terms of inches or degrees. Because of the fact previously noted that, in a standing position, only the base of the body can be considered stationary, it would be extremely difficult and of no practical value to try to determine more exactly how much each point of reference had deviated from plumb alignment.

In the following pages are drawings of the standard posture showing the deep skeletal structures, and the legends indicate which ones coincide with the points of reference. For comparison, beside each drawing is a photograph showing a subject whose alignment approaches closely that of the standard posture.

The detailed explanations which follow are as simple as possible. A section is written with respect to each part of the body for the purpose of presenting what seems to the authors a reasonable and logical explanation of "ideal" alignment.

LOWER EXTREMITY

As illustrated in the following pages, the line of reference in side view passes slightly in front of the ankle joint, slightly in front of the center of the knee joint, and slightly behind the center of the hip joint. The forward curve in the femur permits this relationship of the knee and hip joints to the line of reference.

Since there is no obvious division of the body into anterior and posterior portions, the conclusions regarding the relationship of the line of reference to the body are based on an analysis of what constitutes a stable position of the joints of the lower extremity in standing.

The bony structures of the human body are designed to support and transmit superimposed weight. From a mechanical standpoint, it might be logical to assume that a line of gravity should pass through the centers of the weight-bearing joints of the extremities. It might also be logical to assume that it should pass through the apex of an arch at the base of support. However, from the standpoint of body mechanics, an "on-center" position is not a stable one. It can be held only momentarily in the presence of normal external stresses. The gravity line in a "normal" posture has been described by some* as coinciding with the centers of these joints, but interestingly enough they also acknowledge that the position can be held only momentarily.

The normal limitation of joint motion in certain directions has a postural significance in relation to the stability of the body in the standing position. Dorsi-flexion at the ankle with the knee straight is normally about 10° to 15°. This means that standing barefoot, with feet nearly parallel, the lower leg does not sway forward on the foot more than

* Fick, Braune, and Fisher, according to Steindler.

about 10°. The knee joint has up to 10° hyper-extension. In standing, then, the femur and lower leg relationship will not exceed 10° of postural deviation backward. The hip joint, also, has about 10° hyperextension and, in standing, the joint motion of the pelvis on the femur is restricted to about 10° of postural deviation forward.

When the center of the knee joint coincides with the plane through the gravity line there is equal tendency for the joint to flex or to hyperextend. The slightest force exerted in either direction will cause it to move "off-center". If the body must call on muscular effort at all times to resist knee flexion, for example, there is an unnecessary expenditure of muscular effort. To off-set this necessity, the center of the knee-joint moves slightly behind the line of gravity for stability in standing. (See figs. 5 and 7.)

If the knee joint moved freely backward, this position could not be maintained either without constant muscular effort. Ligamentous structures and strong muscles with tendons that help reinforce the ligaments are the restraining force in this direction. The thrust of body weight above helps to extend the knee joint and ligamentous structures accept the function of counteracting this thrust, all with a minimum of muscular effort.

At the hip joint, the same principles apply but it is forward deviation at this joint that is limited as it is a backward deviation at the knee. The hip joint is most stable when the center of this joint is slightly in front of the gravity line. The strong ligaments that cross the hip joint anteriorly restrict additional forward sway of the pelvis.

There should be careful scrutiny of any manipulation which allows hyperextension of the knee or hip joint, or which excessively stretches such muscles as hamstrings. The normal restraining influence of the ligaments and muscles helps to maintain good postural alignment with a minimum of muscular effort. When muscles and ligaments fail to offer adequate support, the joints exceed their normal range and posture becomes faulty with respect to positions of knee and hip hyperextension.

At the ankle, the line of gravity passes slightly in front of the joint, and the slightly forward deviation of the body is checked by the restraining tension of strong posterior muscles and ligaments. In this relationship to the ankle joint the line of gravity also passes approximately through the apex of the arch, designated laterally by the calcaneo-cuboid joint. (See fig. 7.)

PELVIS

In the side view of the standard posture, the pelvis illustrated is a composite of male and female pelves, and shows an average in regard to shape, length of sacrum, coccyx, and other measurements.

The relation of the pelvis to the line of reference is determined to a great extent by the relationship of this structure to the hip joint. Since the side-view line of reference represents the plane passing slightly behind the hip joint, the pelvis will be intersected through the acetabulum. It is necessary to state what is considered a neutral position of the pelvis in describing the standard posture, and this one point of reference through the pelvis is not sufficient because the pelvis tilts forward or backward about the axis that passes through the hip joints.

Because of structural variations of the pelvis, it appears almost impossible to say that any designated point anteriorly is on the same horizontal plane as a posterior landmark when the pelvis is in a neutral position. The anterior superior spine and the posterior superior spine of the ilium are approximately in that position, however.

The neutral position used as standard by some anatomists* is that in which the anterior superior spines and the symphysis pubis are in the same vertical plane. To the authors of this text, such a position of the pelvis is most acceptable as a neutral position in regard to the standard alignment in the upright posture. It is logical from the standpoint of the action of muscles attached to these two points. The rectus abdominis with its attachment on the pubis extends upward to the sternum, and the sartorius and the tensor fascia lata with their attachments on the anterior superior spines, extend downward to the thigh. In the neutral position these opposing groups of muscles have essentially an equal mechanical advantage in a straight line of pull.

* J. C. Boileau Grant: Method of Anatomy, The Williams & Wilkins Co., 1948. Appleton, Hamilton and Simon: Surface and Radiological Anatomy, The Williams & Wilkins Co., 1949.

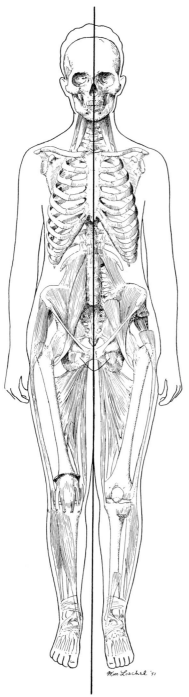

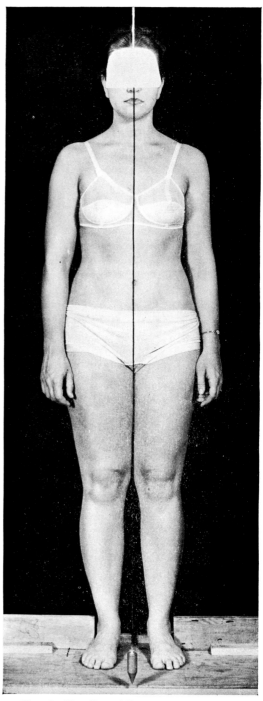

FIG. 1. Standard Posture, Front View

The line of reference coincides with the median plane of the body.

FIG. 2. Excellent Alignment, Front View

The plumb line coincides with the midline of the body. From the standpoint of segmental alignment in this subject the position of the feet and knees is slightly faulty. The feet show slight pronation and the knees slight knock-knee.

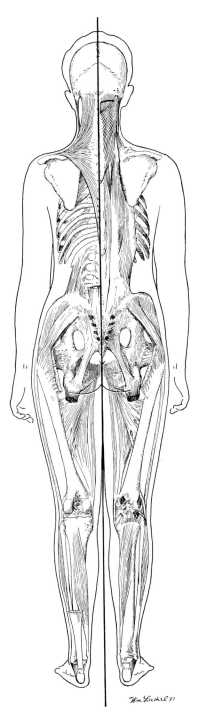

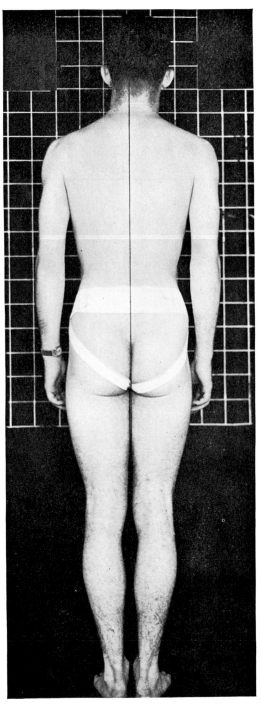

FIG. 3. Standard Posture, Back View

In back view, as in front view, the line of reference coincides with the median plane of the body.

FIG. 4. Excellent Alignment, Back View

In this subject the plumb line coincides with the midline of the body except that the upper trunk and head deviate slightly to the right.

(This is the same subject as seen in fig. 6)

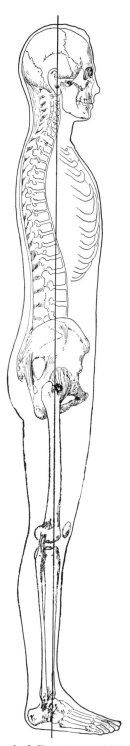

Slightly posterior to the apex of the coronal suture.

Through the external auditory meatus.
Through the dens or odontoid process of the axis.
Through the bodies of the cervical vertebrae.

Through the bodies of the lumbar vertebrae.

Through the sacral promontory.

Slightly posterior to the center of the hip joint.

Slightly anterior to the center of the knee joint.

Slightly anterior to the lateral malleolus.
Through the calcaneo-cuboid joint.

FIG. 5. Anatomical Structures which Coincide with
the Line of Reference

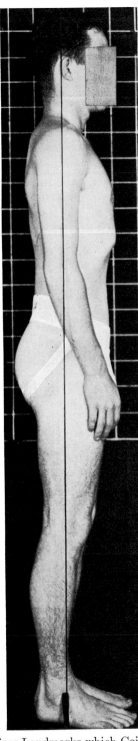

Through the lobe of the ear.

Through the shoulder joint (providing the arms hang in normal alignment in relation to the thorax).

Approximately midway between front and back of the chest.

Approximately midway between the back and the abdomen.

Approximately through the greater trochanter of the femur. *Posterior Extension*

Slightly anterior to a midline through the knee.

Extension

Slightly anterior to the lateral malleolus.

Fig. 6. Surface Landmarks which Coincide with the Plumb Line. (This subject shows excellent alignment except that the head is slightly forward.)

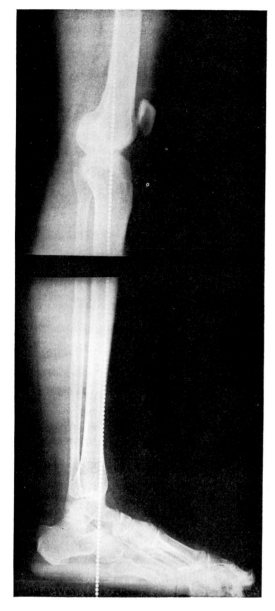

FIG. 7

The above illustration shows the relationship of the plumb line to the bones of the foot and lower leg, with the subject standing in a position of good alignment. The beaded metal plumb line was suspended beside the subject when the x-ray was taken. Two x-ray films were in position for the single exposure.

FEET—A CONSIDERATION OF WHETHER OR NOT THEY SHOULD BE PARALLEL

In the standard posture, the position of the feet is given as one in which the heels are separated about three inches, and the forepart of each foot is abducted about 8 to 10 degrees from the midline.

This position of the feet refers only to the static and barefoot position. Elevation of the heels and motion affect the foot position. Since the usual standing position for the average individual is one in which the heels are elevated to some degree, it is more important to understand the foot position in relation to heel height. A rather detailed analysis follows. The conclusion drawn from the material presented is that a parallel position of the feet is indicated for the average individual who wears an average heel.

Much has been written about the angle of the feet in relation to the standing position and to gait. There is a wealth of information available regarding the mechanics of the foot and the relationship to other joints of the lower extremity. However, the interpretation of the mechanics in terms of postural significance seems inadequate.

A degree of out-toeing used to be considered correct for both standing and walking. Various authorities, in the field of Orthopedic Surgery especially, have observed that such a position of the feet is conducive to a weakening of the structures of the foot, and have advised that the feet should be parallel in walking. Some advise, also, that the feet should be parallel in the standing position, but there is more variance in this opinion.

Morton*, who is considered by many as an outstanding authority on the feet, advocates, however, a degree of out-toeing. He states that "Physiological analysis indicates that the most natural position of the feet in standing is that in which the heels are together while the forepart of the feet are separated sufficiently to give proper security to the lateral balance of the body. Thus the angle of out-toeing should be about 30 to 40 degrees in order that the width of the area of foot contact be equal to its length. This angle is diminished during locomotion."

* Morton, Dudley J.: The Human Foot, Columbia University Press, 1935.

On the assumption that the most natural position of the feet in standing is with heels together, the argument that there should be out-toeing for lateral stability is convincing. The authors question the basic assumption and regard the natural standing position as one in which the feet are separated at the heel as well as at the forepart of the foot. Stability is increased when the base is square rather than tripod. Though separation at the front of the feet with heels together may result in the addition of lateral stability it also results in the loss (proportionately to the angle of separation) of stability in the forward and backward direction. Laterally there are two bases of support so that in any tendency to sway off balance, either may assume full support. In the antero-posterior direction there is, functionally, one base of support and it is not logical to decrease its efficiency in regard to balance, as occurs with the tripod base position.

To further establish the conclusions drawn regarding the position of the feet it is necessary to consider the relationship of the foot to the rest of the lower extremity with particular reference to where, if at all, rotation should occur. It should not occur at the knee joint. On the basis of anatomical construction of the knee joint, there is no rotation in extension. It may be assumed that the axis of the extended knee joint is in a frontal plane, and that it should be so from the standpoint of forward progression as in walking.

Assuming this relationship of the knee joint to the frontal plane, the possibility that outward deviation of the foot should take place from hip joint level is eliminated since rotation of the hip would affect the knee.

This makes the question of whether there should be rotation of the foot into an out-toe position dependent on an analysis of the relationship of the foot and ankle to the lower leg. As a movement, rotation is not present in the ankle joint. In regard to position, the question is whether the ankle joint, like the knee joint, is in a frontal plane. The answer, according to anatomists, is that it is not but that it is slightly oblique. The line of obliquity is such that it extends from slightly anterior at the medial malleolus to slightly posterior at the lateral malleolus. The angle at which the axis of the ankle joint deviates from the frontal plane suggests that the foot is normally in a position of slight abduction (or out-toeing) in relation to the lower leg. But the position of the axis of the joint also suggests that movement about this axis would result in the

foot moving inward as it moved upward, and outward as it moved downward. Functionally, this does not occur.

Passive or active movements of the foot reveal that the foot tends to abduct and evert in full dorsi-flexion, and that the range of motion in plantar-flexion is more free in adduction than in abduction. In other words, the foot tends to move *out* as it moves upward, and *in* as it moves downward, the reverse of the direction suggested by the axis of ankle joint motion.

The answer to much of the discussion regarding proper foot position in standing and walking revolves, then, about the following:

1. What is the anatomical relationship of the foot to the leg in standing barefoot as compared with standing in shoes with heels?
2. How does speed of progression affect foot position?

The relationship of the foot to the lower leg must be analyzed with regard to the arc of motion and the position within that arc of motion which is the equivalent of the upright position, with and without heels.

According to Whitman,[*] "Extreme abduction is attained in the attitude of dorsal flexion, its extent being about one-half that of adduction; the entire range of motion between the two extremes being about 45 degrees." If this figure is acceptable the degree of abduction of each foot in the fully dorsi-flexed position is about 15 degrees and that of adduction about 30 degrees in the plantar flexed position. If an angle of 30 to 40 degrees between the feet were permitted in the standing position, the feet would have assumed the position of maximum abduction. The movement of abduction is so closely related to pronation (or eversion) that many authorities say these terms may be considered synonymous. This being true, the question of what constitutes a good standing position in relation to the degree of abduction must necessarily involve a consideration of the degree of pronation that is advisable.

The foot in full abduction actually represents, in the weight-bearing position, also a position of potentially full pronation. Since the standing position is not one in which the foot is fully dorsi-flexed on the lower leg, it does not follow that a position of full abduction is anatomically correct. From the

[*] Whitman, Royal: A Treatise on Orthopaedic Surgery, Lea & Febiger, 1919, p. 660.

standpoint of stress and strain on the foot itself, a position which permits full pronation is most inadvisable.

As abduction and pronation are related, so also are adduction and supination (or inversion). As abduction is normally related to dorsi-flexion, so adduction is closely related to plantar flexion.

It is difficult, if not impossible, to determine exactly what degree of abduction or adduction of the foot corresponds with each degree of dorsal or plantar flexion. The two are not necessarily so correlated that an exact relationship exists. If it may be assumed, however, that the movement from abduction in the dorsi-flexed position to adduction in the plantar flexed position is relatively uniform, then the following analysis may give a clue to the natural position of the feet in relation to the height of heel.

For purposes of computing the relationship, the normal ranges of motion are stated as follows:

Dorsi-flexion.... ...... 15 degrees above
                                        right angle
Plantar flexion........ 60 degrees below
                                        right angle
Abduction (in dorsi-
    flexion).............. 15 degrees
Adduction (in plantar
    flexion).............. 30 degrees

The full range of antero-posterior motion, i.e., 15 degrees dorsal flexion plus 60 degrees plantar flexion, is 75 degrees. In lateral motion, it is 15 degrees (abduction) plus 30 degrees (adduction) or 45 degrees. The following table then gives the degree of abduction or adduction that corresponds with each 15 degrees change from dorsal to plantar flexion of the foot.

DORSAL TO PLANTAR FLEXION	ABDUCTION TO ADDUCTION
15° dorsal flexion	15° abduction
90° neutral................	9° abduction
15° plantar flexion........	3° adduction
30° plantar flexion........	12° adduction
45° plantar flexion........	21° adduction
60° plantar flexion........	30° adduction

When wearing shoes with heels, the standing position represents varying degrees of plantar flexion of the foot based on the heel height as related to foot length, or more precisely, to the length of the foot from the heel to the ball of the foot. It would be futile to make an effort to compute the degree of out-toeing that corresponds to each heel height according to foot length.

It should be sufficient to know that as the heel height is increased the tendency toward parallel position or in-toeing increases.

The relationship of heel height to out-toeing or in-toeing of the foot is interestingly analogous to the relationship of the foot to standing, walking, and running. Standing barefoot, a slight degree of out-toeing is natural. Standing with heels raised or walking fast, the feet tend to become parallel. In running, the heels do not contact the ground, and the weight is borne on the anterior part of the foot entirely. There is then a tendency for the print of the forefoot to show in-toeing.

CHAPTER II
POSTURAL FAULTS

Most of the specific faults dealt with in this chapter are clearly defined through the use of illustrations and descriptive legends. A few basic terms, however, need to be defined.

Definitions

The word *deviation* is used throughout the book in general discussion as meaning a departure from an accepted form, but in this chapter it will be used specifically to denote deviations of the body from the standard vertical alignment. The term is modified by the words *anterior* (or forward), *posterior* (or backward), *right*, and *left*, and is used in connection with plumb-alignment. The common terms of lordosis, kyphosis, hyperextended knees, etc. denote deviations in alignment with reference to segments of the body.

Tilt refers to rotation about a horizontal axis and is used in relation to the pelvis and the head. An *anterior pelvic tilt* is one in which the anterior-superior spines move down and forward. A *posterior pelvic tilt* is one in which the anterior-superior spines move up and backward. A *lateral pelvic tilt* is not a pure tilt because there is no single axis about which the movement occurs, but is the position of the pelvis when it is lower on one side than on the other, i.e., down on the right or left.

Rotation refers to rotation about a vertical axis. Specifically it is used in relation to the pelvis, head, trunk, thorax, or extremities. In relation to the extremities, the usual terms of internal (or inward) and external (or outward) rotation apply. In relation to the head the rotation is named right or left by the direction in which the face turns, that is, the face toward right is rotation right. Rotation of the pelvis or thorax is referred to as *clockwise* or *counterclockwise*. Considering a horizontal plane through the pelvis, or thorax, and looking at it as if from above, a rotation forward on the right is counter-clockwise rotation; a rotation forward on the left is clockwise rotation.

Lordosis is an increased anterior curve of the spine, usually found in the lumbar region and associated with an anterior pelvic tilt. If used without any modifying word, it refers to lumbar lordosis. Occasionally it is seen in the dorsal spine. The cervical spine position is similar to a lordosis in cases of round upper back with compensatory forward position of the head.

Kyphosis is an increased posterior curve which is usually found in the dorsal spine but which may be present in the lumbar spine. If used without any modification, the word refers to a dorsal kyphosis; if referring to the low back, it is called a lumbar kyphosis. A lumbar kyphosis is usually associated with a posterior pelvic tilt.

Round shoulders refers to a position of abduction of the scapulae and a forward position of the shoulders. It is usually associated with "hollow-chest" position.

Round upper back refers to an increased posterior curve in the dorsal spine. It is the same as a dorsal kyphosis, and is usually associated with a depressed chest. (The round shoulders may be thought of as a curve in the horizontal plane while a round upper back as an increased curve in the vertical plane.)

The gluteal fold or buttocks fold is the horizontal crease between the buttock and the thigh; the gluteo-femoral crease.

The gluteal cleft or cleft of the buttocks is the vertical crease between the right and left buttocks.

Leg refers to the lower extremity. The part between the knee and hip will be referred to as the thigh, and the part below the knee (including the foot) as the lower leg unless otherwise specified.

Arm refers to the upper extremity, with the upper arm, forearm, and hand as the separate parts of the arm.

Knock-knee is a condition in which the knees come together while the feet are apart.

Bow-legs is an alignment of the legs in which there is an outward bowing of the bones of the legs.

The terms *valgus* and *varus* in relation to the knees (i.e., genu valgum and genu varum) are purposely not used in this text.*

Postural bow-legs refers to an alignment of the legs in which the appearance of bow-legs results from standing with the knees in hyperextension and internal rotation, without any true bowing of the bones of the legs. (See fig. 41.)

---

* By derivation, valgus refers to bow-legged, and varus to knock-kneed. Textbooks on Orthopedic Surgery use the terms to describe the opposite. Stedman's Medical Dictionary recognizes that the terms have been mutually reversed in meaning.

Pronation refers to a poition of the foot in which the weight in standing is borne on the inner side of the foot; also eversion or valgus.

Supination refers to a position of the foot in which the weight in standing is borne on the outer side of the foot; also inversion or varus.

The photographs shown in this text specifically illustrate various faults of alignment. The photographs of most of the adult male subjects, while they illustrate specific faults, do not necessarily reflect the typical fault of that individual because these subjects were tod to assume what they considered their best stalding posture. The adult female subjects asd the children, on the other hand, were told to take their natural standing position. The latter is the preferred procedure, and the more indicative of the usual postural alignment of the individual.

ILLUSTRATIONS

FIGURES 8–54

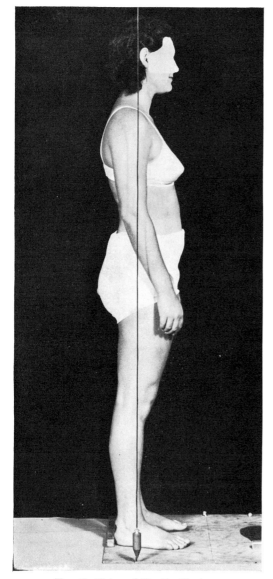

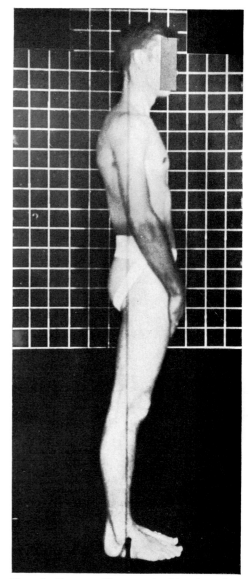

FIG. 8. Relaxed Faulty Posture

This subject shows a typical relaxed faulty posture suggestive of "resting against the ligaments". The knees and upper trunk deviate backward, the pelvis and head forward. The shoulders and upper back are slightly rounded. Fig. 9 is similar but the postural deviations are more pronounced.

FIG. 9. Posture Characterized by Anterior Deviation of the Pelvis

In this type of posture there is hyperextension of the hip joints in contrast to the hip flexion associated with a lordosis posture. The gluteal fold is clearly visible and the buttock is flattened against the posterior thigh instead of being prominent as seen in fig. 10. The lumbar curve is short and shallow; the dorsal curve extends into the lumbar region producing a long kyphosis.

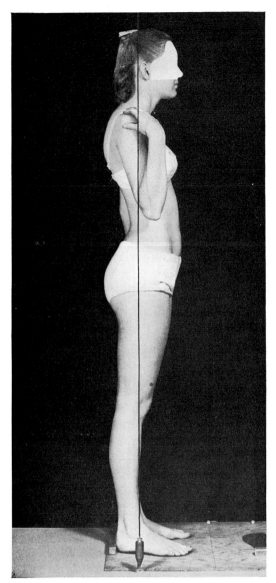

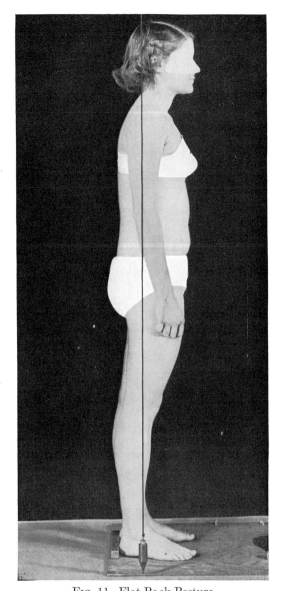

FIG. 10 Lordosis-Kyphosis Posture

This subject shows a very faulty posture with increased forward curve in the lumbar spine, increased backward curve in the dorsal spine, a forward head and hyperextension of the knees.

FIG. 11. Flat Back Posture

This subject shows a decrease in the normal anterior curve of the low back and a posterior tilt of the pelvis resulting in hip joint hyperextension. The knees are hyperextended and the head is forward.

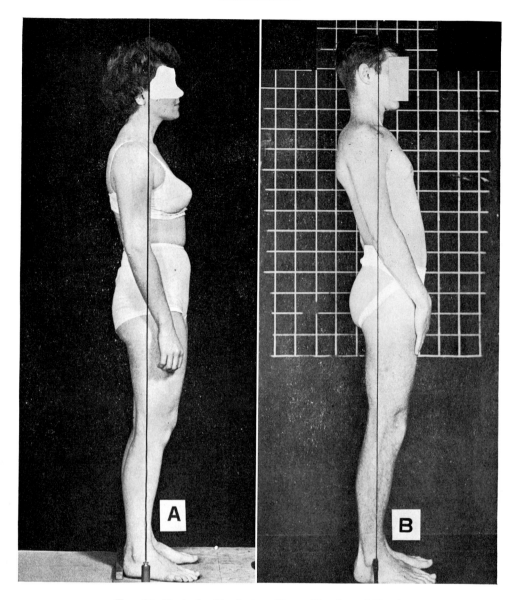

FIG. 12. Posterior Deviation, Upper Trunk and Head

This type of posture is seen rather infrequently. Fig. A shows a relaxed position with a mild posterior deviation of the upper part of the body. Observe that the head is forward from the standpoint of segmental alignment even though it is posterior in relation to the plumb line.

Fig. B shows a more marked posterior deviation and is apparently holding the position with some effort. In each case the knees are slightly flexed to bring the weight of the lower part of the body somewhat forward for balance.

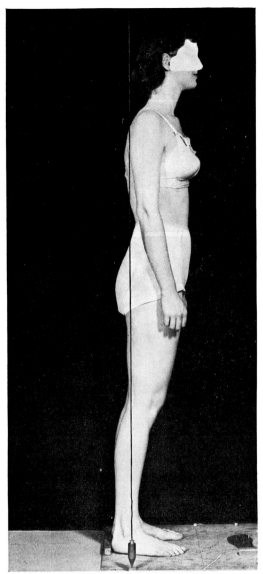

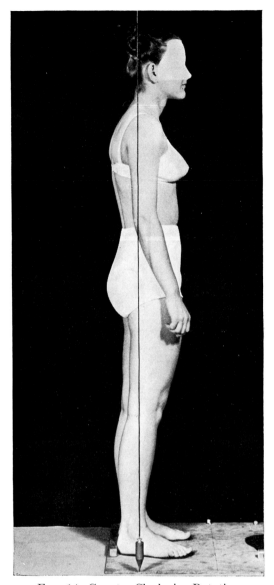

FIG. 13. Anterior Deviation, Marked

The above subject shows a posture which is very faulty in relation to the plumb line. The body weight is carried forward over the balls of the feet. Knees are necessarily slightly flexed in cases of this type deviation. The over-all segmental alignment does not appear very faulty, however. This type of fault is more common in tall slender individuals than in persons of other type build.

FIG. 14. Counter-Clockwise Rotation

This subject shows a counter-clockwise rotation of the body from the ankles to the cervical region.

The deviation of the body from the plumb line appears different from the right and left sides in subjects which have such rotation. The body is anterior from the plumb line as seen from the right, but would show fairly good alignment from the left. From both sides the head would appear forward.

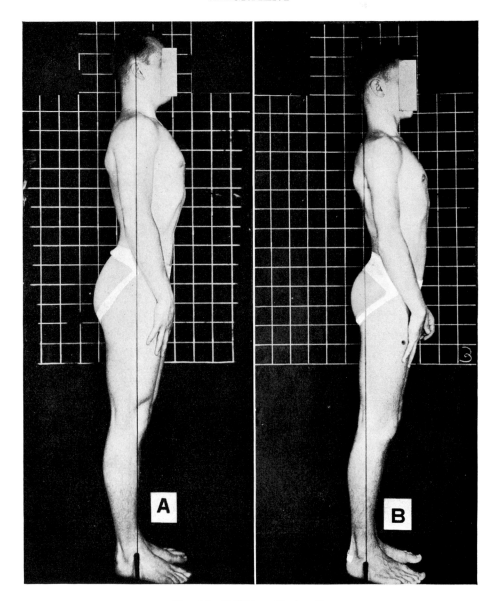

FIG. 15. "Military Posture"

Fig. A shows a moderately faulty "military" type posture, and fig. B shows one that is markedly faulty. An elevated chest and lordosis are apparent in both. Fig. A is quite good in relation to the plumb line, but B is very faulty. (It is not quite as faulty as might at first be observed because the plumb line is slightly posterior at the base.) Evidence of foot strain is present in fig. B. Faulty alignment of this type throws undue stress on the feet.

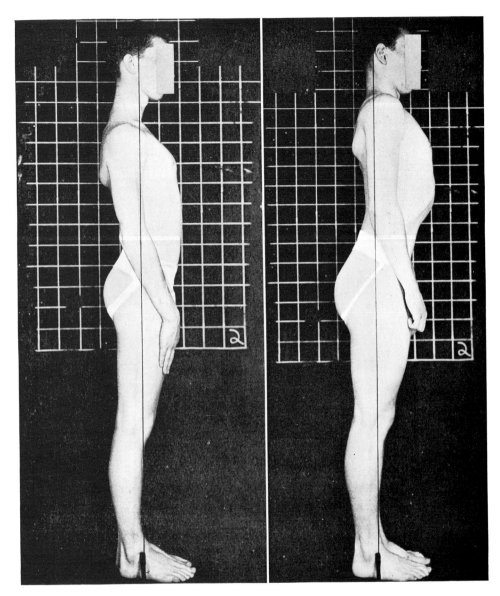

FIG. 16.   "Exaggerated" Posture   FIG. 17.

The above figures represent similar postural problems. Each shows a sweeping lordosis and a distorted appearance of the upper back. Fig. 16 appears more at ease, and shows what is probably quite an habitual position. Fig. 17 is more tense. Although the chest is elevated and chin retracted forcibly, the upper trunk and head are deviated forward because of flexion of the trunk on the thighs.

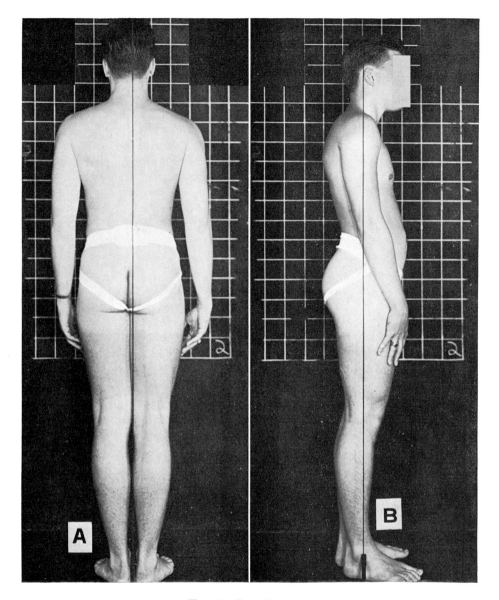

Fig. 18. Poor Posture

This subject is an example of posture which appears good in back view but is very faulty in side view.

The side view shows a lordosis-kyphosis posture which has marked segmental faults, yet in which the anterior and posterior deviations compensate for each other so that the plumb alignment is quite good. It is interesting to note that the contour of the abdominal wall almost duplicates the curve of the low back.

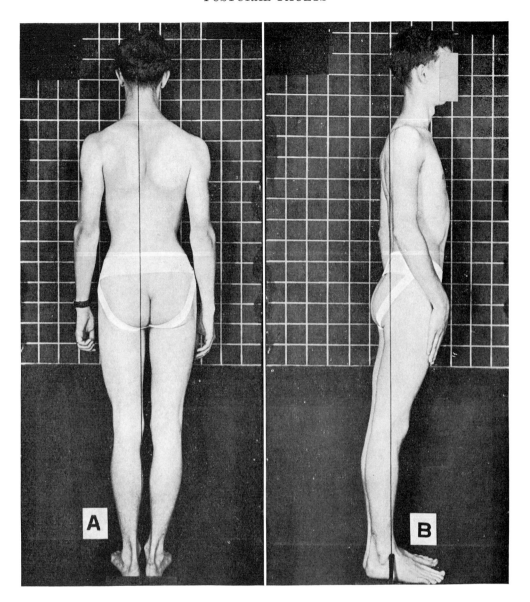

FIG. 19. Very Poor Posture

This subject shows a posture which is faulty in both side and back views. The back view shows a marked deviation of the body to the right of the plumb line, a high right hip, and a low right shoulder.

In side view the plumb alignment is worse than the segmental alignment. The knees are posterior, the pelvis, trunk, and head are markedly anterior. Segmentally the antero-posterior curves of the spine are only slightly exaggerated. The knees, however, are quite hyperextended.

This type of posture might well result from the effort to follow such misguided but common admonitions as "Throw your shoulders back", "Stand with your weight over the balls of your feet".

The result in this subject is so much forward deviation of the trunk and head that the posture is most unstable and requires a good deal of muscular effort to maintain balance.

In uniform or civilian dress, an individual with this type of fault might appear as one with quite good posture.

In this, as in Fig. 15B, the feet show evidence of strain.

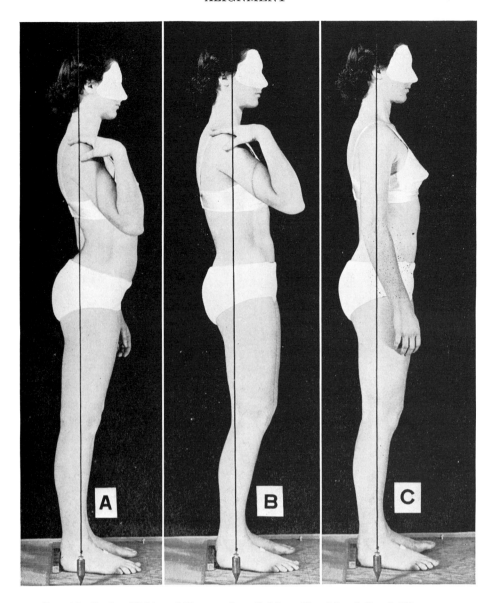

FIG. 20. Faulty Habits of Posture in a Subject Capable of Good Alignment

The three illustrations above, taken on the same date, show two faulty positions and a position of good alignment. The subject stated that she used to stand in a position of extreme sway-back, as illustrated in fig. A, and that her mother constantly tried to get her to correct the fault. In her endeavor to correct she assumed the posture shown in fig. B. This had become her more habitual way of standing at the time she was first seen by the authors. Fig. C shows that the subject is capable of assuming an excellent position. (This is the same subject as shown in fig. 42.)

This series indicates to some extent the faults resulting from a lack of good instruction. It is interesting to compare fig. A with fig. 144D.

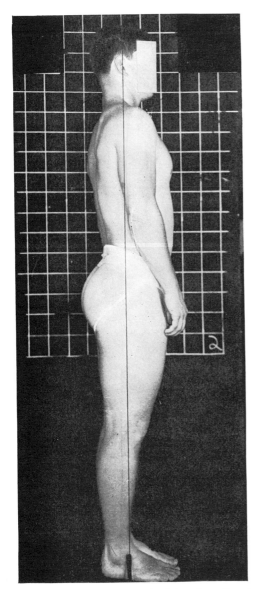

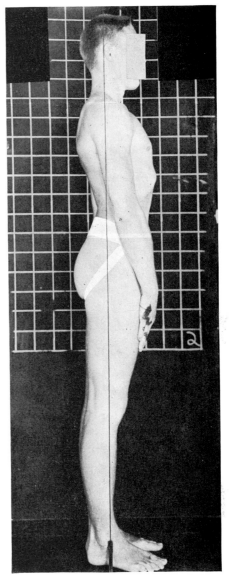

FIG. 21. Posture Characterized by Low Lumbar Lordosis

This subject shows a marked anterior pelvic tilt with increased angulation of the spine in the lumbosacral region. There is evidence of counter-clockwise rotation of the trunk.

FIG. 22. Posture Characterized by High Lumbar Lordosis

This subject shows a high and rather marked lordosis. The pelvis and lumbar spine are inclined forward to the level of about the second lumbar vertebra. Above this level there is a sharp deviation backward resulting in a lordosis which is angular rather than smoothly curved like the one seen in fig. 10.

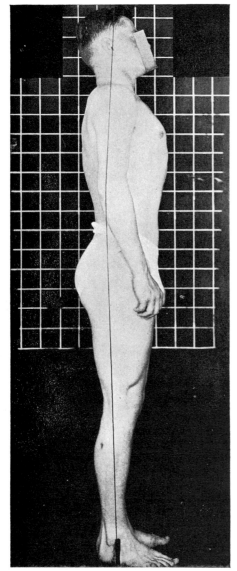

FIG. 23. Head, Posterior Tilt

In this subject the head tilts backward and there is hyperextension of the cervical spine. The chest and shoulders are held high.

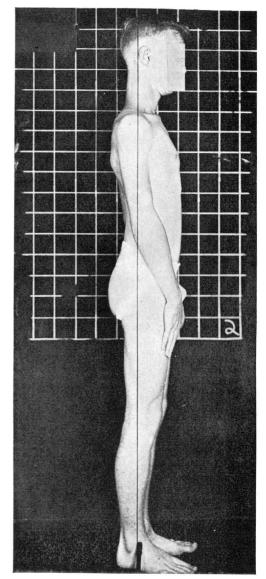

FIG. 24. Head, Anterior Tilt

In this figure the head is tilted forward and the cervical spine is in flexion.

A posture in which the normal anterior curve of the cervical spine tends to reverse, as it does in this subject, is most unusual. According to Gray "flexion is arrested just beyond the point where the cervical convexity is straightened. . . ." and this subject shows what appears to be maximum flexion.

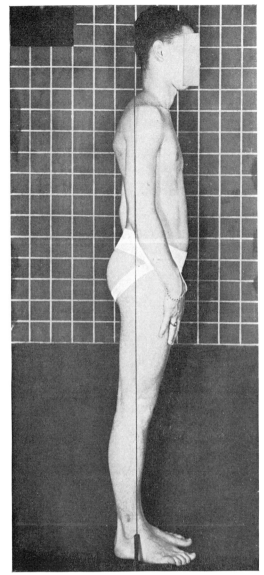

FIG. 25. Forward Head with Attempted Correction

In this picture the subject is apparently trying to correct what is basically a forward head position.

The curve of the neck begins in a typical way in the low cervical region, but a sharp angulation occurs at about the 6th cervical vertebra. Above this level the curve seems very much decreased. The chin is pressed against the front of the throat. This distorted rather than corrected position of the neck results from a failure to correct the related faulty posture of the pelvis and upper trunk.

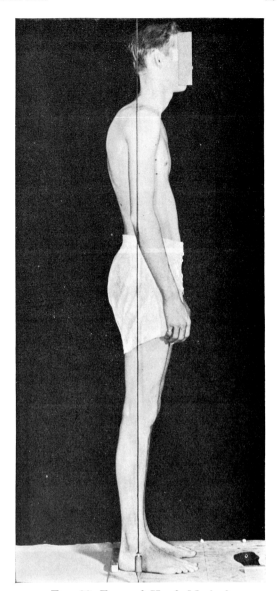

FIG. 26. Forward Head, Marked

This subject shows an extremely faulty alignment of the neck and dorsal spine. The degree of deformity in the dorsal spine is suggestive of an epiphysitis. This patient was treated for pain in the posterior neck and occipital region.

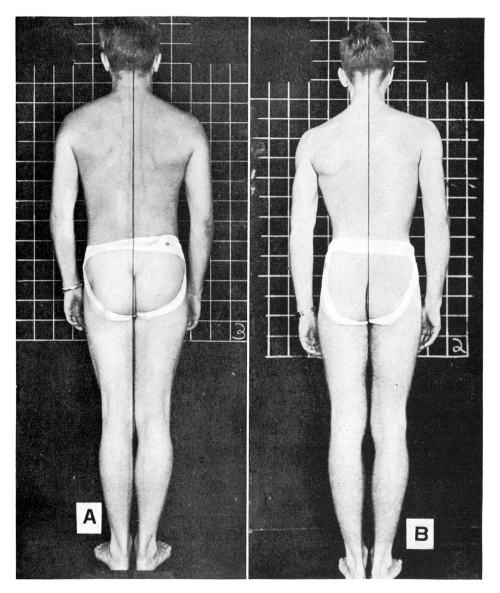

FIG. 27. Handedness Patterns

Each of the above figures illustrates a typical pattern of posture as related to handedness. In fig. A the right shoulder is lower than the left, the pelvis is deviated slightly toward the right, and the right hip appears slightly higher than the left. This pattern is typical of right handed people. Usually there is a slight deviation of the spine toward the left and the left foot is more pronated than the right. Fig. B shows the opposite pattern which is typical of left handed individuals. Usually, however, the low shoulder is not quite as marked while the high hip is more marked than this figure shows.

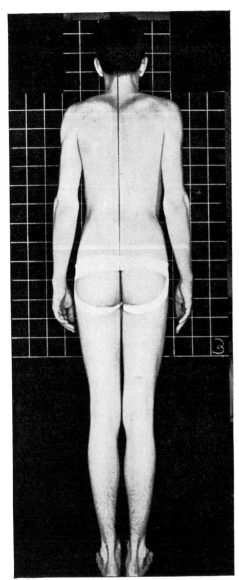 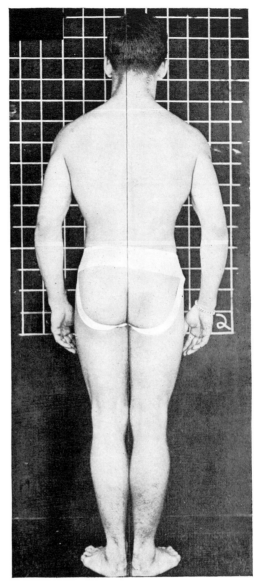

Fig. 28. Shoulders, Elevated

In this figure both shoulders are elevated with the right slightly higher than the left.

The scapulae are somewhat adducted.

The upper trapezius and other shoulder elevators are in a state of contraction.

Fig. 29. Shoulders, Depressed

In this picture the shoulders slope downward sharply, accentuating their natural broadness. The marked abduction of the scapulae also contributes to this effect of broadness.

Strengthening the trapezius muscle, particularly the upper part, tends to correct this type of fault.

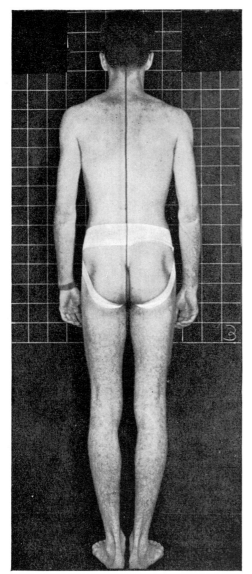

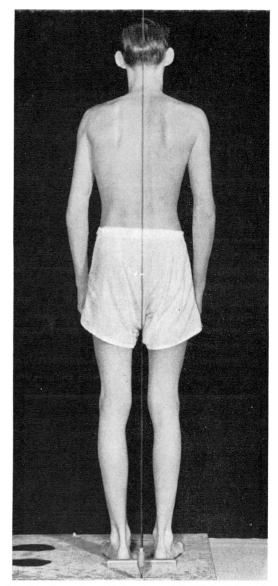

FIG. 30. Scapulae, Good Position

This picture illustrates a natural position of the scapulae.

They lie flat against the thorax and no angle or border is unduly prominent. Their position is not distorted by unusual muscular development or misdirected efforts at postural correction.

FIG. 31. Scapulae, Abduction with Slight Elevation

In this subject, both scapulae are abducted, the left one more than the right. There seems to be no rotation of the scapulae, but they are slightly elevated. This kind of elevation goes with round shoulders and round upper back. For side view of this subject see fig. 26.

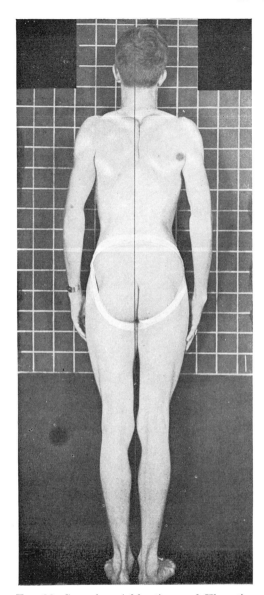

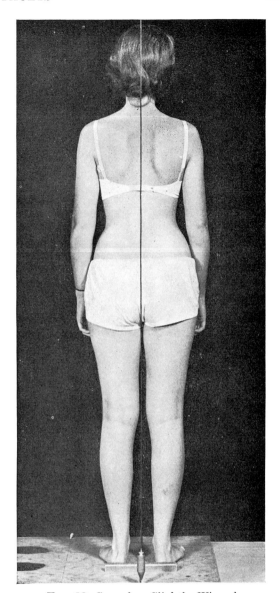

FIG. 32. Scapulae, Adduction and Elevation

The scapulae in this picture are completely adducted and considerably elevated.

The position illustrated is obviously held by voluntary effort, but when this habit has persisted for some time the scapulae do not return to normal position when the subject tries to relax.

This position is the inevitable end-result of persisting in the military practice of "bracing" the shoulders back.

FIG. 33. Scapulae, Slightly Winged

In this figure, the scapulae are fairly prominent. They do not lie flat against the thorax.

In this particular case, there is slight serratus anterior weakness. A strikingly similar appearance is seen in individuals who have a flattening of the dorsal spine.

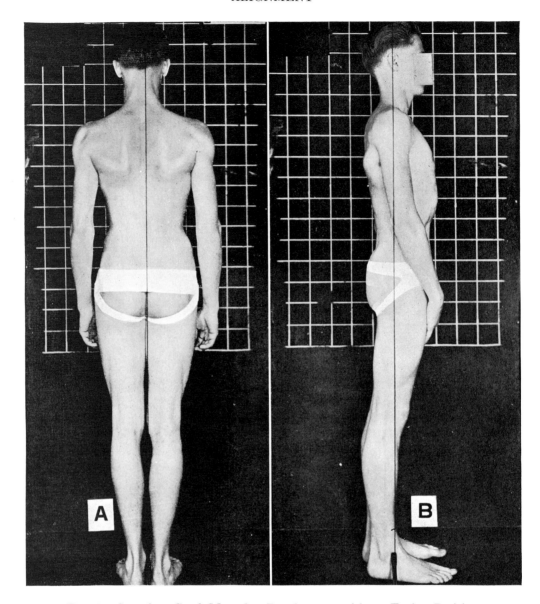

FIG. 34. Scapulae, Good Muscular Development without Faulty Position

In back view this subject shows a well developed musculature of the shoulder girdle with the scapulae in good position.

The teres major muscle is clearly seen extending from the axillary border of the scapula to the arm, forming the bulge seen in the arm pit.

In side view of the same subject the bulk of this muscle is very apparent, and the profile of the upper back appears somewhat distorted by this muscle mass.

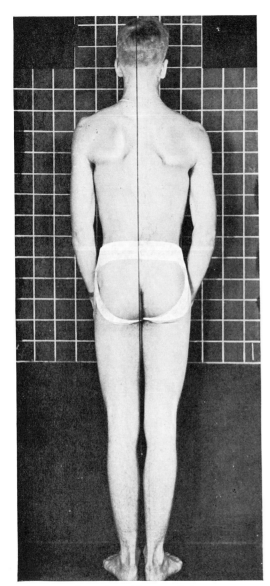

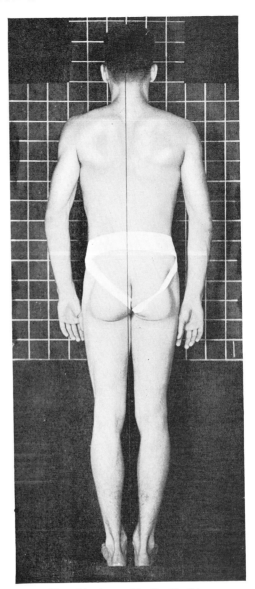

FIG. 35. Scapulae, Abnormal Appearance

This subject shows abnormal development of some of the scapular muscles with a faulty position of the scapulae.

The teres major and rhomboids which show clearly, form a V at the inferior angle. The scapula is tilted so that the axillary border is more nearly horizontal than normal. The appearance suggests marked weakness of either the serratus anterior or the trapezius or both.

FIG. 36. Arms, Faulty Position

In this figure the arms hang in a position of internal rotation. The palms of the hand face almost directly backward instead of toward the sides of the body.

The position of the arms suggests over-development and some tightness in the internal rotator group of muscles. The teres major is one of this group, and its over-development is quite apparent.

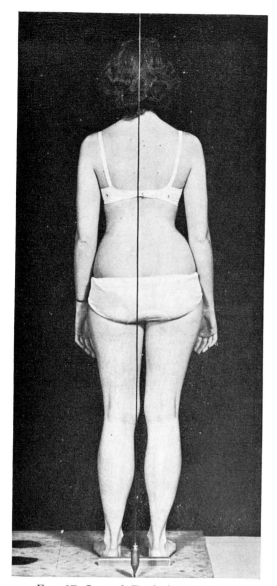

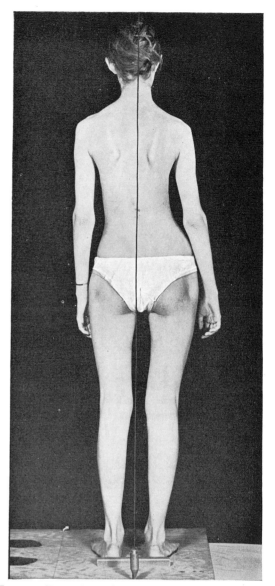

FIG. 37. Lateral Deviation of Pelvis

This subject shows a marked deviation of the pelvis to the right of the plumb line giving the appearance of a high hip on the right. The shoulders are level. There is a slight dorso-lumbar curve to the left, though this is not apparent in the illustration because the spine is not marked.

FIG. 38. Lateral Deviation of Pelvis with Scoliosis

The posture of this subject resembles that in the previous figure but the shoulders and scapulae are not level. They are lower on the right, and the subject has a fairly marked left dorso-lumbar scoliosis.

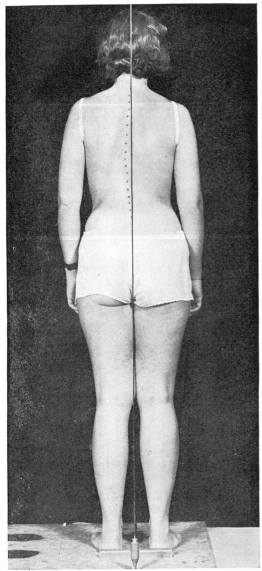

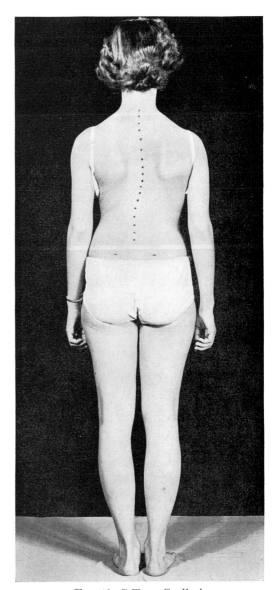

Fig. 39. C-Type Scoliosis without Pelvic Deviation

In this subject the pelvic deviation is negligible, and the pelvis is level but there is a left C-curve of the spine and the right shoulder is lower than the left.

Fig. 40. S-Type Scoliosis

In this subject there is a right dorsal, left lumbar curve with deviation of the pelvis toward the left. This subject is an acrobatic dancer and shows a pattern which the authors have seen quite frequently among those engaged in this profession.

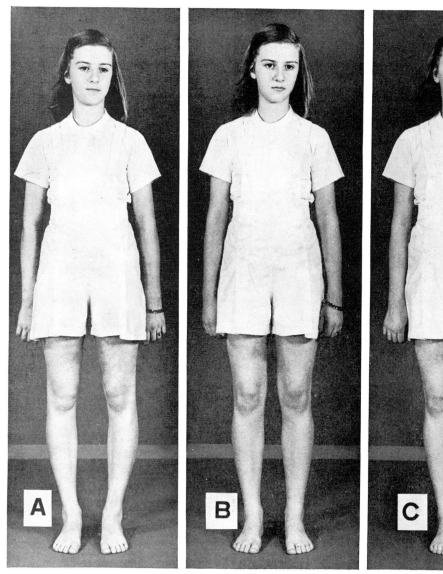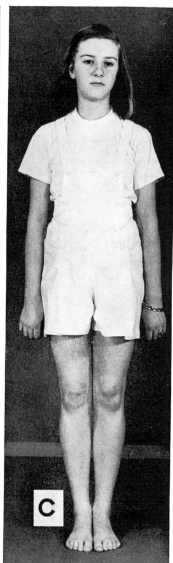

FIG. 41. Postural Bow Legs, Child

In A the subject has thrust the knees back and allowed them to internally rotate and bow outward slightly. The feet have been allowed to pronate.

In B the feet have not been moved from the position in A, the knees have been brought into a position of normal extension, and the postural bowing of the legs disappears as hyperextension and the accompanying internal rotation are corrected.

C shows a simple check on bony alignment. If knees touch when feet are together, the alignment is good and there is no evidence of any structural fault.

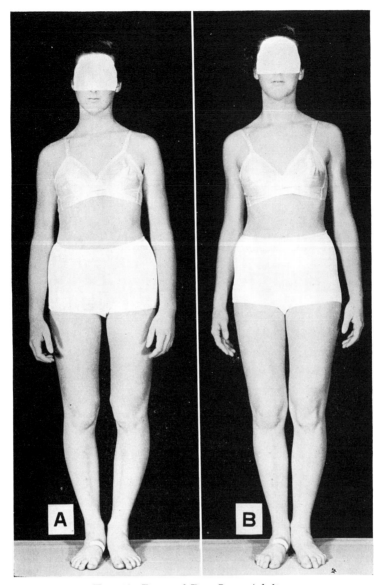

FIG. 42. Postural Bow Legs, Adult

Fig. A shows a position of postural bow-legs which has been habitual for a period of years. In this case there is an associated marked pronation of the feet. Fig. B shows an effort to correct the faulty position. Although not complete, there is evidence of the possibility of good correction. This subject is very flexible (see fig. 20) and probably is capable of a greater degree of correction than most young adults who have had this persistent fault.

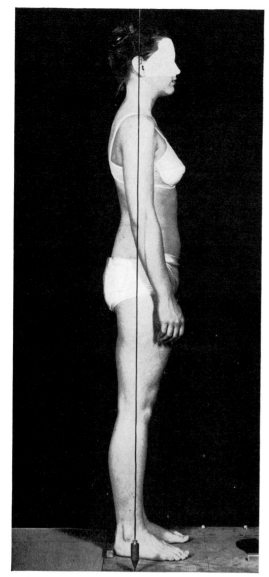

FIG. 43. Knees, Good Alignment

In good alignment of the knees in side view the plumb line passes slightly anterior to a midline through the knee. (This is the same subject who is seen in the front view in fig. 2.)

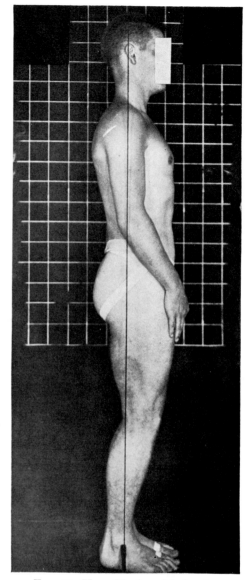

FIG. 44. Knee Flexion, Moderate

Flexion of the knees is seen less frequently than hyperextension in cases of faulty posture. The flexed position requires constant muscular effort by the quadriceps. Knee flexion in standing may result from hip flexor tightness. When hip flexors are tight there must be compensatory alignment faults of the knees or the low back or both. The degree of lordosis that results if the knees are kept straight is decreased if the knees are flexed.

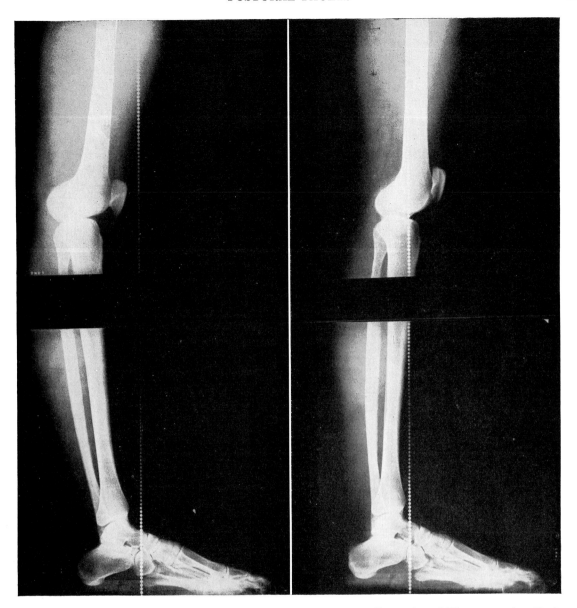

FIG. 45. X-ray of Knee in Marked Hyperextension

This x-ray is of a subject who had a habit of standing in hyperextension as a child. The plumb line was suspended in line with the standard base point while the x-ray was taken. The cassettes were placed between the lower legs and thighs during the single x-ray exposure.

FIG. 46. Correction of Hyperextension Fault

The above x-ray is of the same subject shown in fig. 45. As an adult she has attempted to correct her hyperextension fault. The alignment through the knee joint and femur are very good, but the tibia and fibula show evidence of posterior bowing.

Compare with fig. 7.

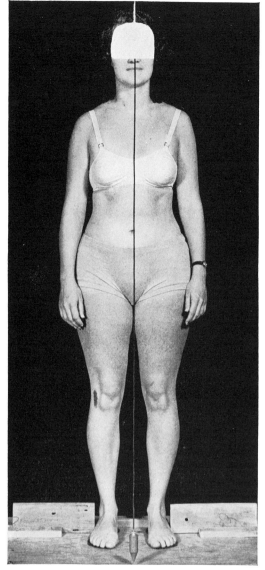

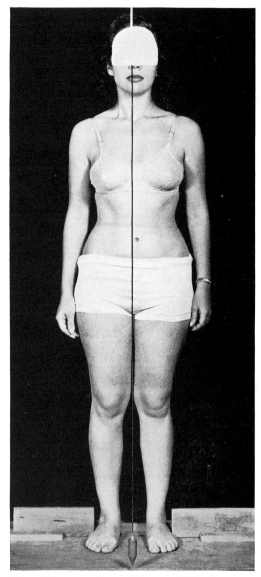

FIG. 47. Pronation of Feet and Internal Rotation
of Femurs

The distance between the lateral malleolus and
the foot board indicates a moderate pronation of
the feet, and the position of the kneecaps indicates
a moderate degree of internal rotation.

FIG. 48. Pronation of Feet and Knock-knees

The feet are moderately pronated; there is slight
knock-knee position, but no internal or external
rotation.

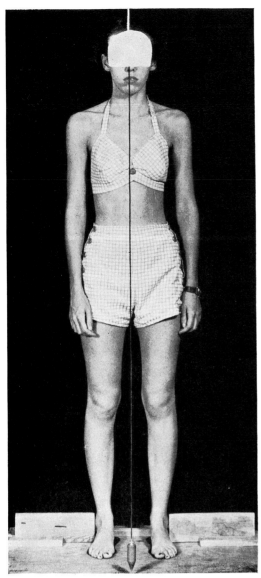

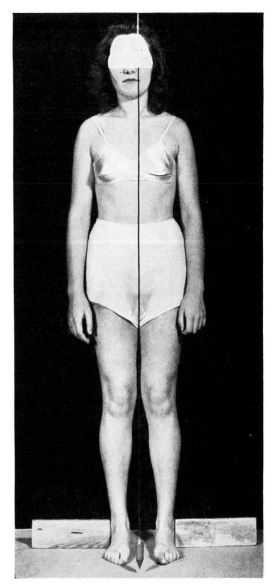

FIG. 49. Feet Good, Knees Faulty

The alignment of the feet is very good but there is internal rotation of the femurs as indicated by the position of the patella. This type fault is harder to correct by use of shoe corrections than one in which pronation accompanies the internal rotation.

FIG. 50. Supinated Feet

In the figure above, the weight is borne on the outer borders of the feet, and the long arches are higher than nornal.

The perpendicular foot-board touches the lateral malleolus, but is not in contact with the outer border of the sole of the foot.

The position shown is the natural posture of this subject's feet, but the anterior tibial muscles show so clearly that it appears as if an effort were being made to invert the feet.

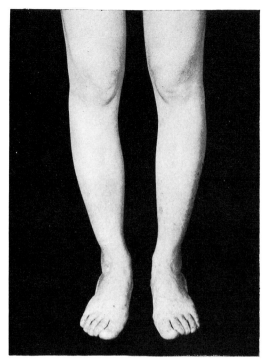

FIG. 51

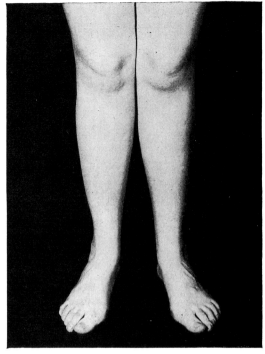

FIG. 53

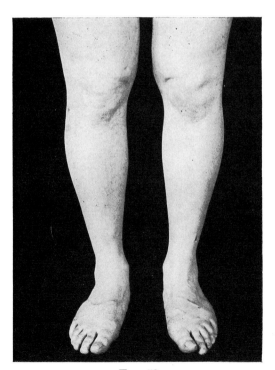

FIG. 52

FIG. 51. Pronation with Flattening of Arches

This figure shows marked pronation of both feet, flattening of the longitudinal arches, and the position of the toes indicates that the metatarsal arches are depressed. The faulty position of the feet and knees results in a torsional strain in which the long muscles of the foot (which have their origin on the tibia and fibula) are subjected to undue strain.

FIG. 52. Flat Longitudinal Arches

Although the longitudinal arches are very flat, there is less pronation and less associated faulty mechanics of the knee position in this subject than illustrated in the previous figure.

FIG. 53. Beginning Hallux Valgus

This subject shows a beginning hallux valgus in which the big toe deviates toward the midline of the foot.

In later stages there tends to be a bony enlargement on the inner side of the base of the big toe, resulting in a "bunion".

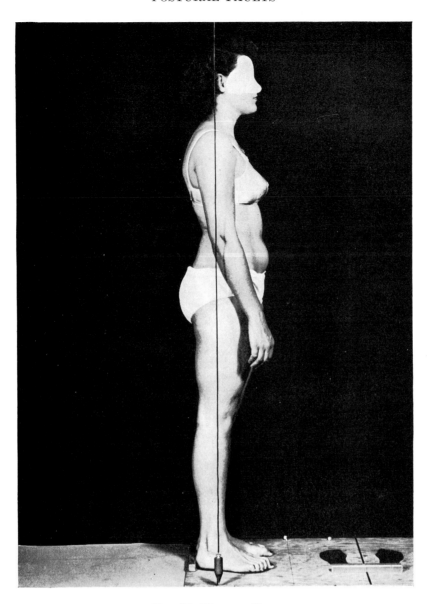

FIG. 54. Hammer Toes

This subject shows marked hammer toes with
tightness of the toe extensors, the tendons of which
are clearly visible.

PART II

MOBILITY

CHAPTER III

JOINT AND MUSCLE ANALYSIS AND RELATION TO POSTURE

A disturbance of muscle balance, particularly if it involves major muscles of the lower extremities and trunk, will be reflected in some form of postural deviation. Muscles that are tight tend to pull the body segments to which they are attached out of line. Muscles that are weak allow deviation of the body segments by their lack of support.

Just as initial weakness or tightness of muscles may cause faulty alignment, so faulty alignment may give rise to adaptive weakness or tightness. The appearance of the fault is the same in either case, making it impossible to distinguish cause and effect in this regard in established postural faults.

Movements which strengthen or weaken muscles are the means by which muscle balance is maintained or altered. When an imbalance exists, exercises are used as therapeutic measures for the purpose of restoring muscle balance.

An analysis of the muscle and joint actions occurring in various exercise movements, and an analysis of the muscle imbalances present in various types of faulty posture are essential to an understanding of the use of therapeutic exercise in correction of postural faults.

This chapter deals with exercises and postural positions involving, primarily, the relationship of the pelvis to the lower extremities and spine, because the position of the pelvis is regarded as the keynote in postural alignment. It aims to show the relationship of the muscle actions which occur in exercise movements to the muscle imbalances present in faulty alignment in order to provide a sound basis for prescribing therapeutic exercises. One should not prescribe for postural correction those exercises which tend to increase the strength of already strong muscles, nor those which tend to put undue load or tension on weak muscles.

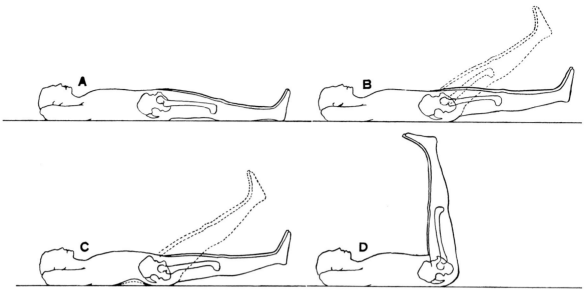

FIG. 55. Movements Involved in Double Leg-raising

Double leg-raising is a combination of two movements; a fixation of the pelvis by the abdominal muscles, and flexion of the thighs on the pelvis by the hip flexors.

A shows the first phase of the movement, a posterior tilting of the pelvis done by the abdominal muscles. In this position the pelvis acts as a base for the pull of the hip flexor muscles.

B shows leg-raising performed by an individual whose abdominal muscles are strong enough to hold the pelvis in a *posterior tilt* throughout the whole movement.

C. The pelvis is in a position of *anterior tilt*. This position occurs when the strength of abdominal muscles is not sufficient to prevent the weight of the legs from tilting the pelvis forward. The average child or female adult cannot prevent such a tilt from occurring at the beginning of the leg-raising movement. The dotted line shows that, as the legs are raised, the curve in the back tends to be decreased.

D shows the position of the pelvis in a completed leg-raising movement. As the legs approach the vertical, the pelvis is pulled into a posterior tilt by tension of the hamstring muscles as well as by action of the abdominals. In the position illustrated the legs have slightly passed the vertical and the pelvis has

about completed its range of posterior tilt. This might be the final position of the movement shohw in either B or C.

In leg-raising the greatest effort is demanded from both the hip flexor and abdominal muscles when the legs are nearly horizontal. Here the resistance of gravity is maximal, and neither group of muscles is in a position of good mechanical advantage. Usually the hip flexors succeed in flexing the thighs on the pelvis, but in most cases the abdominal muscles are unable to keep the pelvis tilted posteriorly. When the weight of the legs tilts the pelvis anteriorly it means that the pull of the abdominal muscles has been overcome and the muscles themselves have been subjected to undue stretch and strain.

Because of decreased gravitational resistance and a gradually increasing mechanical advantage, the ability of the abdominals to fix the pelvis is greater as the legs approach the vertical. As this happens the danger of strain is lessened.

In abdominal muscle weakness, leg-raising is not a safe movement to be used as an exercise. Even more harmful is the practice of asking an individual to try to hold his legs a few inches above the floor for a specified number of seconds, as is done sometimes in giving achievement tests. For a discussion of abdominal tests and exercises see pp. 79–83 and p. 128.

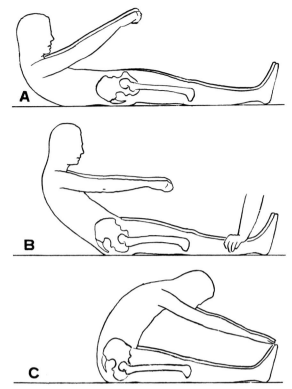

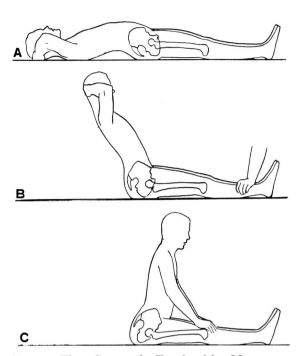

FIG. 56. Three Stages of a Trunk-raising Movement
with Flexion of the Spine

In A the action is chiefly *trunk flexion*, bringing
the sternum and pubis closer to each other by raising
the upper trunk and tilting the pelvis backward. The
active muscles are the abdominals. The hip flexors
are elongated by the posterior tilting of the pelvis
with the legs straight.

In B the position of trunk flexion is maintained
by the abdominals while the movement of *flexion of
the pelvis on the thighs* is performed by the hip flexors.
During this phase of the movement the legs may
need to be held down by an assistant to give better
fixation for the action of the hip flexors and to
counteract the weight of the trunk.

In C the subject has completed the normal range
of this trunk-raising movement. After the upper
trunk has passed the perpendicular, gravity helps
in the action.

FIG. 57. Three Stages of a Trunk-raising Movement
with Hyperextension of the Spine

When done as illustrated above, trunk-raising is
primarily a *hip flexion* movement throughout, and is
accomplished by the hip flexors. Fixation of the legs
by an assistant is needed from the beginning of the
movement until the weight of the trunk has passed
the perpendicular. This movement can be done by
a person with strong hip flexors even if the abdominal
muscles are paralyzed. Raising the trunk in hyperextension causes an uncomfortable stretch of the
abdominal muscles, especially the rectus abdominis.

A shows the movement beginning with hyperextension of the lumbar spine by the back extensors
and flexion of the pelvis on the thighs by the hip
flexors.

In B the hip flexors have continued to bring the
trunk upward. Gravity is largely responsible for
the hyperextension of the trunk. The abdominals
are on a stretch.

C shows the movement beyond the normal range.
Gravity assists in hip flexion and the stretch on the
abdominals is much reduced. The hyperextension of
the back is due to the action of the back muscles
holding the trunk erect or may be due to shortness
of back extensors.

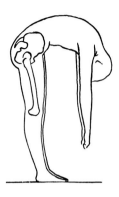

FIG. 58. Hip and Trunk Flexion, Standing

This movement is similar to the one shown in fig. 56C with the addition of a backward deviation of the pelvis. The muscle action differs because of the changed relation to gravity. Hip and trunk flexion are accomplished by gravity and a controlled release by back and hip extensors. The same muscles that gradually lengthen to lower the trunk actively shorten to raise it.

Abdominal and hip flexor muscles are used only if the movement is limited by tightness of posterior muscles and an effort is made to pull downward against such restriction.

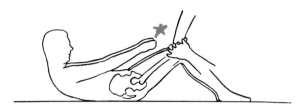

FIG. 59. Hip and Trunk Flexion

This movement is one which is sometimes recommended as a means of testing or exercising abdominal muscles without hip flexor action. The theory is that bending the knees relaxes the hip flexors sufficiently to keep them from acting. Instead, this degree of knee-bend places the hip flexors in a position of good mechanical advantage. The fixation of the legs gives them a good base from which to pull. (To confirm the fact that they do go into action as soon as the abdominals start to flex the trunk, one need only palpate the superficial hip flexors tendons.)

Compare this with fig. 56A in which the hip flexors are at a mechanical disadvantage because they are elongated and without fixation.

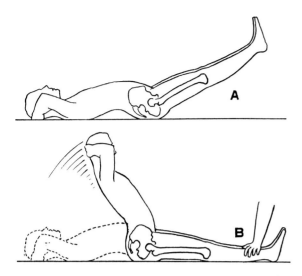

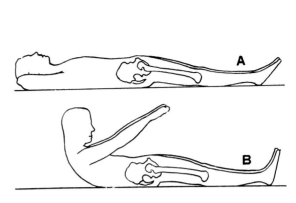

FIG. 60. Leg- and Trunk-raising in Cases of Paralyzed Abdominal Muscles and Strong Hip Flexors

As illustrated in A above, an individual with strong hip flexors can raise both legs even though the abdominal muscles are paralyzed. The subject can complete flexion of the hip joint, but the legs will not be raised through their normal arc because the pelvis has tilted forward. With lack of abdominal muscles there is no fixation of the pelvis on the thorax anteriorly. Fixation in a position of anterior tilt results when the spine locks in hyperextension.

With very weak abdominal muscles and over-developed hip flexors, an individual can come to a sitting position if the legs are held firmly down and the subject is allowed to do the movement quickly, as illustrated in B. The hip flexors initiate the action by flexion of the pelvis on the thighs and pull the hyperextended trunk forward with the aid of momentum.

FIG. 61. Attempted Leg- and Trunk-raising in Cases of Strong Abdominals and Paralyzed Hip Flexors

As illustrated in A, if the hip flexors are paralyzed an individual cannot lift the legs even though the abdominal muscles are strong. The abdominal muscles can have no action on the thigh because none of them crosses the hip joint.

Under normal circumstances the movements of pelvic tilt and hip flexion both occur in double leg-raising. (See discussion, p. 50.) In the absence of hip flexors, only the abdominal action occurs, namely the posterior pelvic tilt.

As shown in B, if hip flexors are paralyzed and the abdominal muscles are strong, an individual can perform only the trunk flexion part of the trunk-raising movement.

The pelvis tilts posteriorly as in the normal initiation of this movement (See fig. 56A) but the lack of hip flexors prevents the initiation of the second phase of the movement, i.e., flexion of the pelvis on the thighs. (See fig. 56B.)

The upper trunk is not lifted as high from the table as in normal trunk flexion because the pelvis tilts posteriorly more than normal due to lack of fixation by the hip flexors. (See last paragraph, p. 55, for discussion of stabilization.)

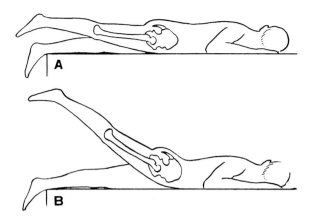

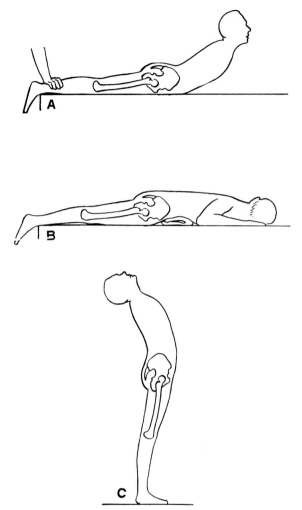

FIG. 62. Movements Involved in Leg-raising
Backward

The movement of leg-raising backward is a combination of two separate motions: one, hyperextension of the hip joint as shown in A, which is limited to about 10 degrees; and, two, pelvic tilt as shown in B. The entire range of motion above the first few degrees is brought about by movement of the pelvis. In the prone position the low back erector spinae muscles are chiefly responsible for this anterior tilting of the pelvis. These muscles are assisted to some extent by the hip flexors on the side of the stationary leg.

The hyperextension of the hip and lumbar spine are initiated almost simultaneously and these two movements are not separate stages in the motion.

If slight tightness exists in hip flexors, there is no range of hyperextension in the hip joint, and all the movement in the direction of leg-raising backward is accomplished by pelvic tilt.

FIG. 63. Hyperextension of Hip Joint,
with or without Hyperextension of Spine

FIG. 63.

As seen in A, the movement of trunk-raising backward combines hyperextension of the lumbar spine and hyperextension of the hip joint. With legs supported, the lower leg is the fixed point from which the action takes place. The hip extensors stabilize the pelvis on the thighs as the low back muscles extend the lumbar spine.

B shows posterior pelvic tilt (i.e., flattening the low back) in the prone position. The movement is accomplished by the hip extensors with assistance from the abdominal muscles. The hip joints are in a position of hyperextension.

C shows a hyperextension of the spine and hip joints in backward bending. The backward displacement of the weight of the upper trunk is counterbalanced by a forward deviation of the pelvis. This brings the hip joint into a position of postural hyperextension. If this movement is done forcefully it is accomplished by the back and hip extensors. Otherwise, the hyperextension of the spine is brought about by gravity. The abdominal muscles and (to a lesser degree) the hip flexors gradually lengthen as the trunk bends back and shorten to raise it to a vertical position.

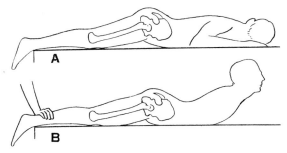

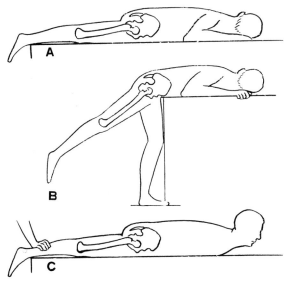

FIG. 64. Attempted Leg- and Trunk-raising in
Cases of Paralyzed Back and Strong
Hip Extensor Muscles

In A, the subject is attempting to lift one leg off
the table. The hip extensors are fully contracted
but the leg cannot be lifted because the back muscles
are unable to stabilize the pelvis. The pelvis has
been tilted posteriorly by the weight of the leg instead of being tilted anteriorly as it would be by
normal back extensor action.

If the pelvis is stabilized by having the trunk
prone on a table and one foot resting on the floor
as shown in B, the hip extensor strength will extend
the leg toward a horizontal position.

In C the subject is attempting trunk-raising backward. He is unable to raise his trunk. The pull of the
hip extensors tips the pelvis posteriorly and flexes
the lumbar spine.

FIG. 65. Attempted Leg- and Trunk-raising
Backward in Cases of Strong Back and
Paralyzed Hip Extensor Muscles

A shows the subject attempting to lift his leg off
the table. The normal tendency of back muscles to
act with hip extensors in this movement results in the
position illustrated. The back contracts to fix the
pelvis on the trunk, but since there is no strength in
the hip extensors, the leg cannot be extended on the
pelvis. The unopposed pull of the back muscles results in hyperextension of the back, and the hip
joint is passively drawn into flexion despite the effort
to extend it.

In B the subject is attempting to raise the trunk
backward. Hyperextension of the spine is completed
but the trunk cannot be lifted as high from the table
as it would be if the hip extensors could stabilize
the pelvis.

Similar examples of the effect of an unstable base
in reducing arc of motion are frequently seen in
paralytic cases. The principle is simple. There is a
limit to the range through which a muscle can pull
the bony part it is moving. Muscles usually work
from a fixed base so that when they shorten they
pull the moving part toward the fixed part. The arc
of motion through which the part travels if the muscle shortens completely is considered the normal
range for that movement. If neither part to which a
muscle is attached is stabilized, each part will move
toward the other as the muscle shortens and neither
part will be moved through its full arc of motion.

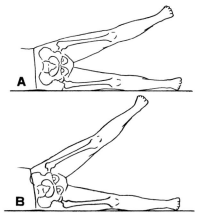

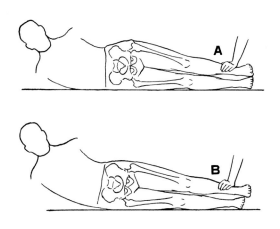

FIG. 66. Movements Involved in Leg-raising
Sideways

Leg-raising sideways involves abduction of the
hip as seen in A and lateral pelvic tilt as seen in B.
The pelvis is tilted upward on the side of the leg
being raised, and downward on the side of the stationary leg. The increase in range of leg raising
seen in B as compared to A is the result of the
lateral pelvic tilt.

On the side of the leg being raised, the hip abductors perform the hip joint motion and, simultaneously, the lateral trunk flexors stabilize the pelvis.
To complete the leg-raising the lateral trunk flexors
"hike" the pelvis upward. On the other side, the
pelvis is pulled downward by the hip abductors,
which act in reverse to pull the pelvis toward the
leg rather than the leg toward the pelvis.

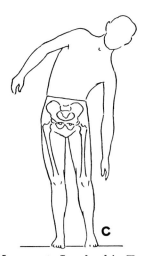

FIG. 67

Trunk-raising sideways consists of lateral trunk
flexion as seen in A accompanied by a tilt of the
pelvis on the legs as seen in B. Translated into terms
of hip joint action the pelvic tilt that accompanies
this trunk-raising toward the left results in abduction of the left hip joint and adduction of the right.
The muscles chiefly responsible for the combined
movements are the lateral trunk flexors on the left,
the left hip abductors, and the right hip adductors.

The legs must be held down to counterbalance the
weight of the trunk, but must not be held so firmly as
to prevent the upper leg from moving slightly downward to accommodate for the displacement downward
of the pelvis on that side.

FIG. 67. Movements Involved in Trunk-raising
and Trunk-bending Sideways

C shows trunk bending sideward from a standing
position. This movement differs from the one in A
chiefly in that gravity causes the lateral flexion instead of opposing it. The right lateral trunk flexors
control the movement. They lengthen gradually to
lower the trunk toward the left and shorten to raise
it. The pelvis shifts to the right to counterbalance
the weight of the upper trunk as it moves to the
left of center. In a forced movement the left lateral
trunk flexors are brought into the action.

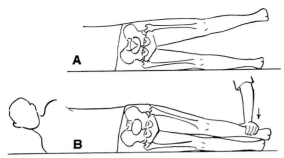

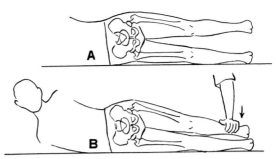

FIG. 68. Attempted Leg- and Trunk-raising Sideways in Cases of Paralyzed Lateral Abdominals and Strong Hip Abductors

In A the subject is unable to raise his leg sideways through its whole arc of motion. The abduction of the thigh has been completed by the hip abductors, but the lateral trunk flexors have been unable to tilt the pelvis upward to complete the range of motion. Due to the weakness of these trunk muscles the weight of the lifted leg tilts the pelvis downward. (See discussion of stabilization, last paragraph p. 55.)

As shown in B the effort to raise the trunk sideways fails completely. The pelvis is tilted downward toward the leg as it should be in this movement, but the thorax cannot be raised sideways toward the pelvis.

FIG. 69. Attempted Leg- and Trunk-raising Sideways in Cases of Strong Lateral Abdominals and Paralyzed Hip Abductors

In A the subject is attempting to raise his leg sideways. The lateral trunk flexors, which normally act to finish this movement, act to initiate it when hip abductor power is inadequate. In tilting the pelvis upward the lateral flexors have drawn the leg into the position illustrated. Although the leg may appear to be abducted, it has actually dropped into a position of maximum adduction at the hip (about 10° beyond neutral). It is held in position by tension of joint structures rather than by hip muscle action.

In B the subject is attempting to do trunk-raising sideways. The lateral trunk flexors are fully contracted but the trunk cannot be lifted through its whole arc of motion because the hip abductors are unable to stabilize the pelvis. (See discussion of stabilization, last paragraph p. 55.) The pelvis has been tilted upward by the weight of the trunk instead of being tilted downward as it would be by normal abductor action.

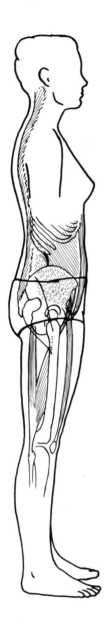 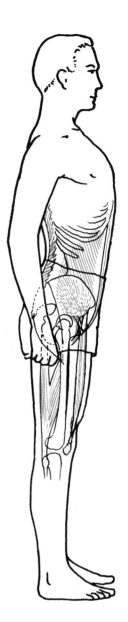

FIG. 70. This figure shows the muscles attached to the pelvis which are chiefly responsible for the maintenance of good alignment of the pelvis in relation to the trunk and legs. The abdominals pull upward anteriorly and the hamstrings downward posteriorly to counterbalance the downward pull of the hip flexors anteriorly and the upward pull of the low back muscles posteriorly.

FIG. 71. In this type of posture the chest is elevated and the pelvis is tilted anteriorly resulting in a lordosis position of the back. The rectus abdominis muscle with attachment on the sternum and pubis is subjected to constant stretch, and persistence in this position results in stretch-weakness of this muscle.

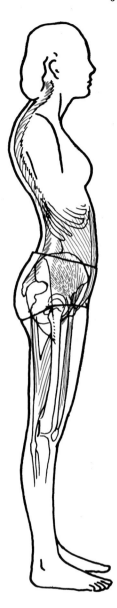

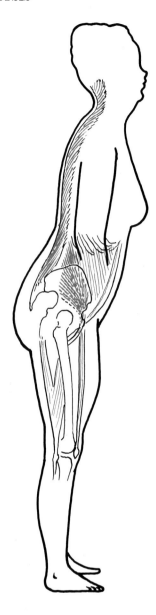

FIG. 72. Lordosis-Kyphosis Posture

This figure shows the pelvis in a position of anterior tilt, the hip joints in flexion, and the low back in hyperextension or lordosis. The low back extensors and hip flexors are tight and strong, while the "lower" abdominals and hamstrings are stretched and weak.

FIG. 73. Postural Hip Flexion

This position results from a backward deviation of the legs and a forward deviation of the upper trunk with a compensatory anterior tilt of the pelvis. The hip joint position is one of flexion, and the trunk is in hyperextension, but to a lesser degree than in fig. 72.

Hip flexors tend to be shorter and back extensors less short than in the lordosis posture at the left.

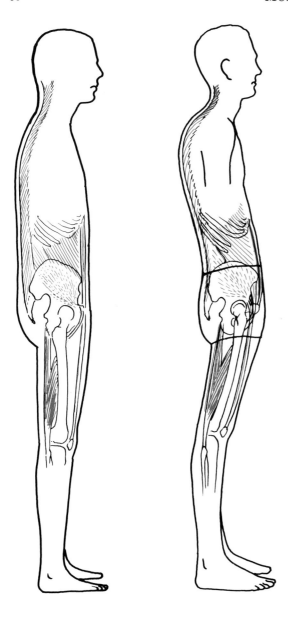

Fig. 74. Flat Back

Fig. 74. shows a "flat back" due to excessive posterior tilt of the pelvis. At the hip joint the pelvis is hyperextended on the thighs. Muscle findings are less constant in this kind of posture than in other types. The most constant finding is a tightness of hamstring muscles which pull the pelvis into posterior tilt. Other common findings are slight weakness of hip flexors, or back extensors, or both. The back muscles may be very strong and inflexible, however, as a result of occupational activity. Abdominal muscles may or may not be strong. Slight knee flexion may be found with this posture due to tightness of the hamstrings.

Fig. 75. Postural Hyperextension of the Hips

In fig. 75 the pelvis and upper end of the legs sway forward in relation to the feet, which remain stationary. This results in hyperextension of the hip joint in the same manner as does raising a leg backward when the pelvis is fixed. The position is called *postural hyperextension of the hip joint*. The pelvis is tilted slightly back. There is no increased anterior curve in the lumbar spine, and hence there is no lordosis. The long curve in the dorso-lumbar region which is due to the backward deviation of the upper trunk is sometimes mistakenly referred to as a lordosis in this type of posture.

This position is limited by, and to a great extent maintained by, the tension of the anterior hip ligaments and of the hip flexor and (external) oblique abdominal muscles. These muscle groups usually show stretch-weakness. The lower back and hamstring muscles are likely to be strong and somewhat short. In the upper trunk the opposite conditions prevail. The upper back muscles show a stretch weakness and the "upper" abdominals are likely to be strong.

FIG. 74   FIG. 75

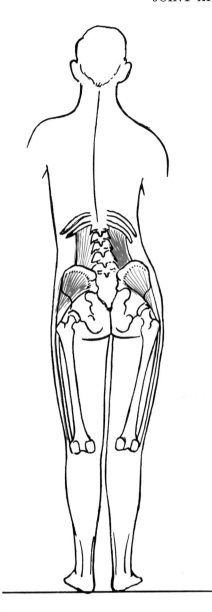

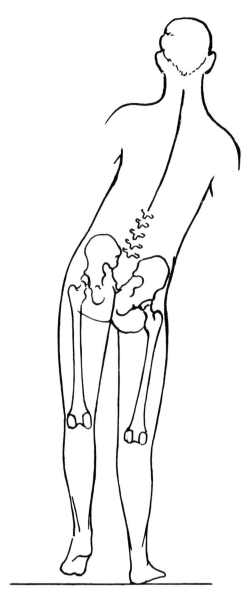

FIG. 76. Postural Adduction, Right Leg

FIG. 77. Gluteus Medius Limp

With a deviation of the pelvis toward the right and a lateral tilt down on the left, the right hip is in adduction and the position is referred to as "postural adduction" of the right leg. In this type posture the right gluteus medius is weaker than the left. The left leg is in a position of "postural abduction" and the left hip abductor group, especially the tensor fascia lata, is often somewhat tight.

This position of the right hip resembles the Trendelenburg sign or gait.

This figure shows the weight-bearing position of abduction assumed by the right leg in an individual who has marked weakness of the right gluteus medius. This is in direct contrast to the hip joint position (fig. 76) in an individual who has mild or moderate weakness of this muscle. Weight of the trunk is thrust toward the affected leg so that the body is balanced over the center of support.

CHAPTER IV
TESTS FOR MUSCLE LENGTH

Muscles have an important role in supporting skeletal structures, but such support must be provided without sacrificing mobility. Thus a muscle must be long enough to permit normal mobility of the joints and must be short enough to contribute effectively to joint stability.

The purpose of muscle length tests is to determine whether the range of joint motion permitted by the muscle length is normal, limited, or excessive. In dealing with problems of faulty body mechanics, there is more concern with muscles which are too tight than with those which are stretched, and more emphasis is placed on the analysis for tightness, hence these tests are often referred to as tests for muscle tightness.

The five muscle-length tests which may be considered essential in postural examination are described and illustrated in this chapter. Accompanying the illustration which shows the normal range of motion expected in these tests in adults is a series of illustrations showing limited or excessive range of motion. Explana-tory legends accompany the illustrations. Included are:

1. The movement of bending forward to touch the finger tips to the toes with knees straight to test for length of posterior muscles including back extensors, hamstrings, and gastroc-soleus.
2. The straight-leg-raising movement to test for hamstring length.
3. The test for tensor fascia lata tightness.
4. The hip extension test for hip flexor tightness.
5. The arm over head extension movement to test for tightness of the adductor and internal rotator group of muscles.

In the line drawings used to illustrate the first three of the foregoing, the same basic figure is used for the normal as for the faulty. It is suggested that the reader make a tracing of the normal figure in each group and use it as an overlay in order to make comparisons of the positions of the spine and pelvis in the series of drawings.

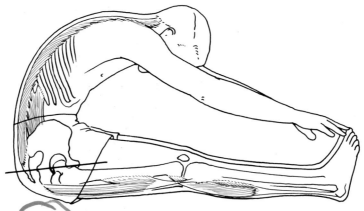

FIG. 78. Normal Length of Back, Hamstring, and Gastroc-Soleus Muscles

Note the line of reference through the pelvis indicating a slight degree of posterior tilt. Note also the contour of the spine.

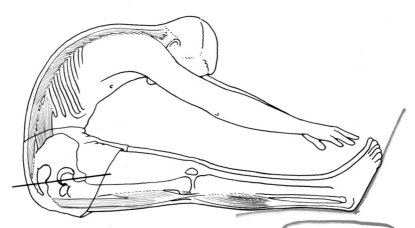

FIG. 79. Normal Length of Back and Hamstring Muscles, Tight Gastroc-Soleus Muscles

This figure is identical with fig. 78 except that the subject cannot pull the feet into dorsi-flexion because of tightness of the plantar-flexor group.

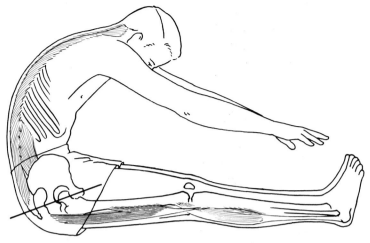

FIG. 80. Normal Length of Back and Gastroc-Soleus Muscles, Tight Hamstring Muscles

Note the line of reference through the pelvis which shows that it is tilted more posteriorly than in the normal subject. Except for the change in pelvic tilt due to hamstring tightness, this figure is identical with fig. 78.

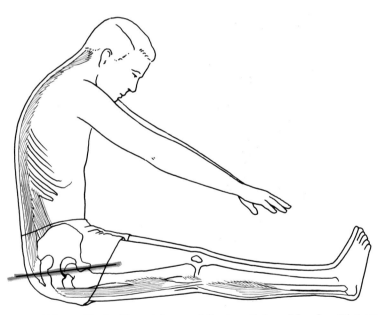

FIG. 81. Normal Length of Upper Back, Hamstring, and Gastroc-Soleus Muscles, Tight Low Back Muscles

This figure is identical with fig. 78 except in the low back region. A tracing of the upper trunk of fig. 78 superimposed upon that in this figure will show that the contour of the spine is exactly the same in both although they appear quite different.

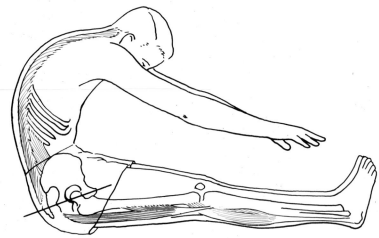

FIG. 82. Stretched Upper Back, Slightly Tight Low Back, Tight Hamstrings, and Normal Length of Gastroc-Soleus Muscles

The excessive flexibility permitted by the stretched upper back muscles does little to counteract the loss of reach caused by low back and hamstring tightness.

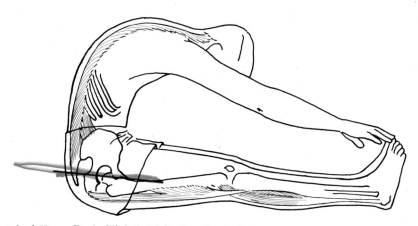

FIG. 83. Stretched Upper Back, Slightly Tight Low Back, Stretched Hamstrings, and Normal Length of Gastroc-Soleus Muscles

Figures 82 and 83 are the same except that the stretched hamstrings have compensated for the tightness of the low back in permitting this subject to touch his toes.

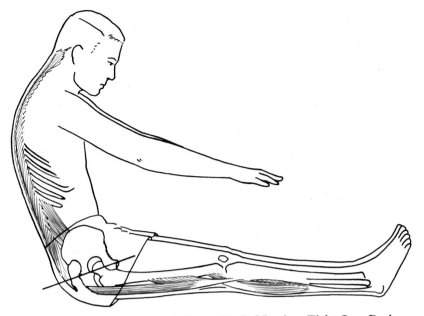

FIG. 84. Normal Length of Upper Back Muscles; Tight Low Back,
Hamstring, and Gastroc-Soleus Muscles

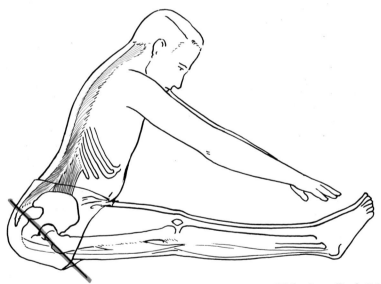

FIG. 85. Normal Length of Upper Back Muscles, Very Tight Low Back Muscles

This figure illustrates forward bending as it is
frequently seen in paralytic cases in which there is
severe involvement of both lower extremities. This
degree of forward tilt of the pelvis on the femur does
not occur if the hamstring muscles have normal tone.

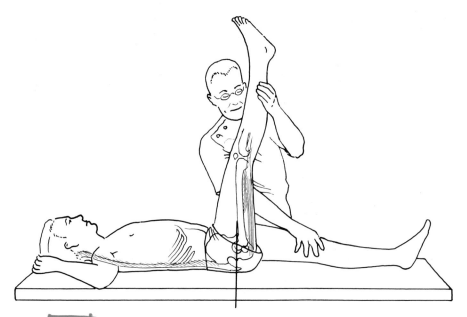

FIG. 86. Normal Length of Right Hamstring, Low Back, and Left Hip Flexor Muscles

The straight leg-raising test is really a combination of hip flexion and slight posterior pelvic tilt. Muscle tightness which restricts either of these movements will affect the test. Range of motion is normal if the angle between the leg and the table is about 80 to 85 degrees with the back flat.

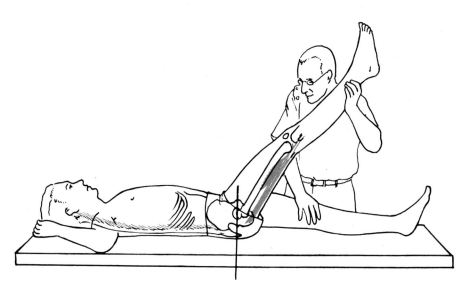

FIG. 87. Tight Right Hamstring Muscles, Normal Length of Low Back and Left Hip Flexor Muscles

This figure shows restriction in the straight-leg-raising test because of hamstring tightness. The low back and the opposite hip flexor muscles have permitted the normal range of posterior pelvic tilt.

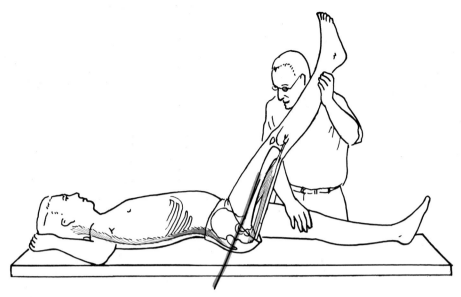

FIG. 88. Normal Length of Right Hamstring Muscles, Tight Low Back and Left Hip Flexor Muscles

The restriction of the straight leg-raising in this figure is due to loss of pelvic tilt, not due to restriction of hip joint motion. The tightness of low back and opposite hip flexor muscles keeps the pelvis in a position of anterior tilt when the left leg is held down on the table. The hip joint is flexed to the same degree as in the normal leg-raising movement, fig. 86.

Pelvis no move

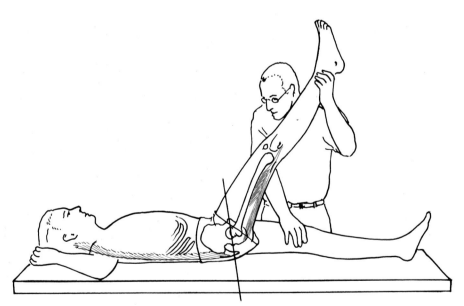

FIG. 89. Tight Right Hamstring Muscles, Stretched Low Back and Left Hip Flexor Muscles

The hamstring tightness in this figure is the same as that seen in fig. 87, but does not appear to be as marked. The pelvis is tilted to the extent that there is a slight lumbar kyphosis. The leg moves through an increased arc of motion because of this increased pelvic tilt.

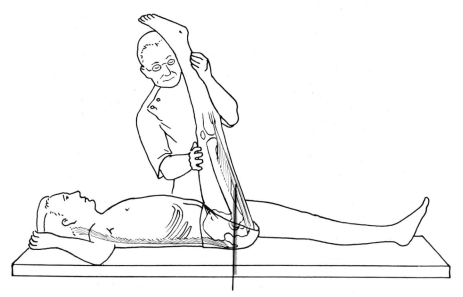

FIG. 90. Stretched Hamstring Muscles Normal Length of Low Back Muscles

The thigh is stabilized anteriorly to prevent knee
flexion. The figure demonstrates an excessive range
of motion.

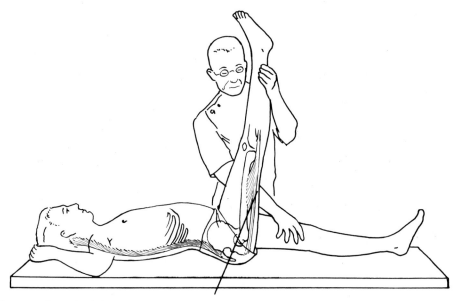

FIG. 91. Stretched Hamstring Muscles, Tight Low Back and Left Hip Flexor Muscles

The range of hip joint motion is identical with
that in fig. 90 but the hamstring stretch is obscured
by the presence of anterior pelvic tilt.

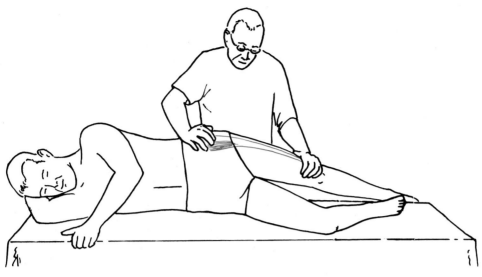

FIG. 92. Normal Length Tensor Fascia Lata*

The normal length of the tensor fascia lata permits the leg to drop in adduction toward the table as illustrated. Observe that the lateral trunk on the under side remains in contact with the table.

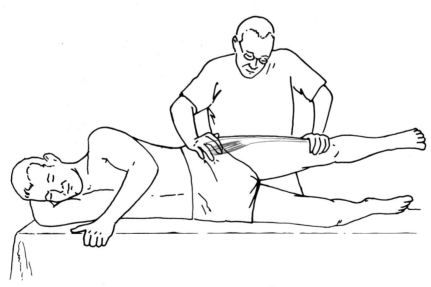

FIG. 93. Tight Tensor Fascia Lata

As seen in this figure, if the leg fails to drop when the pelvis is fixed, it indicates a tightness of the tensor fascia lata and ilio-tibial band.

*[In this text tensor fascia lata refers to the combination of the tensor fasciae latae (or tensor fasciae femoris) muscle and the lateral thigh fascia into which this muscle inserts.]

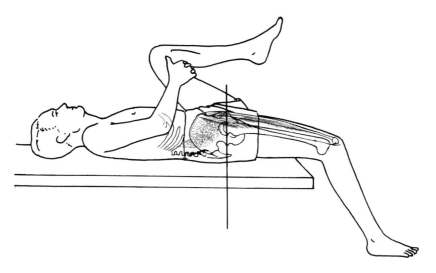

FIG. 94. Normal Length of Hip Flexor Muscles

The ilio-psoas, rectus femoris, tensor fascia lata, and sartorius comprise the hip flexor group. The ability to touch the thigh to the table while the back is held flat, as illustrated, shows normal length of the hip flexor group.

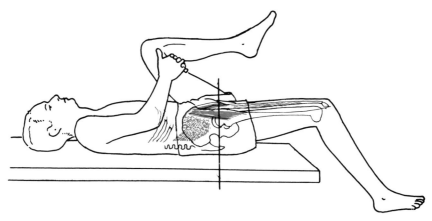

FIG. 95. Tight Hip Flexor Muscles

The inability to bring the thigh down to touch the table indicates hip flexor tightness.

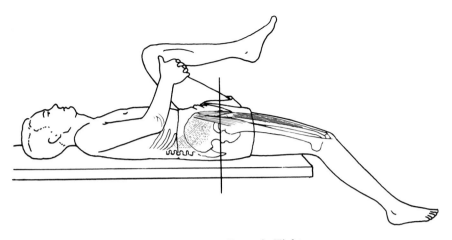

FIG. 96. Rectus Femoris Tightness

If the knee extends as the thigh is brought down to touch the table, there is evidence of rectus femoris tightness. The remaining hip flexors have permitted hip extension, and the tightness of the rectus femoris has been referred to the knee.

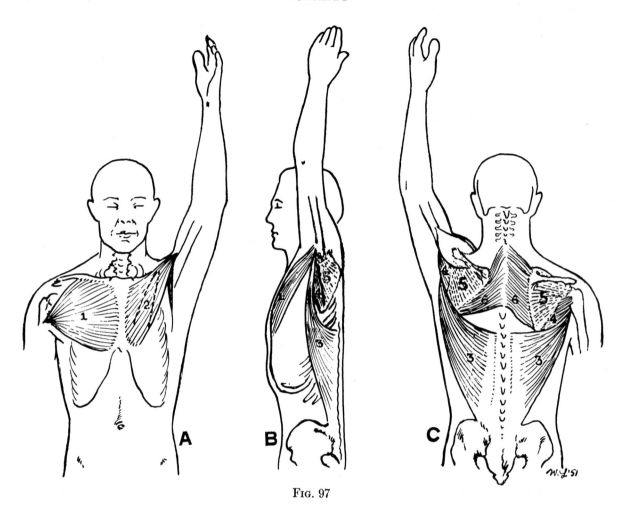

FIG. 97

The illustration above shows the chief muscles
which by their length permit full range of scapulo-
humeral and scapular motion for normal overhead
extension of the arm. The muscles included are: 1)
pectoralis major, 2) pectoralis minor, 3) latissimus
dorsi, 4) teres major, 5) subscapularis, 6) rhomboids.

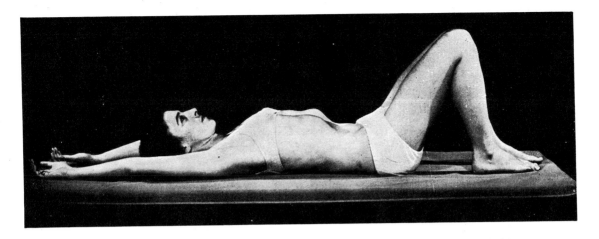

FIG. 98. Test for Normal Length of Adductors and Internal Rotators of the Arm

With the back flat the arms should rest easily on
the table near the head. The knees are bent to insure
holding the back flat on the table.

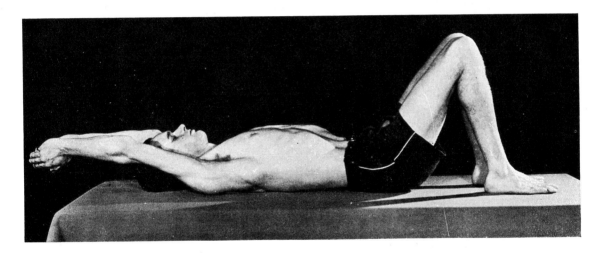

FIG. 99. Tightness of Adductors and Internal Rotators of the Arm

The position of the arms in this subject indicates
moderate tightness of adductor and internal rotator
muscles.

Although it is not an adductor or internal rotator
of the shoulder joint, a tight pectoralis minor may
restrict full overhead extension of the arm by holding the scapula depressed forward. Since tightness
of the minor may be present without noticeable
tightness of the other muscles, it is advisable to
check separately for this. The subject lies supine, as

illustrated, but with arms down at the sides. Except
in cases of a fixed kyphosis, the shoulders will lie
flat on the table if no tightness is present in the
minor. If the shoulders are tilted forward, the examiner presses downward on them and gauges the
amount of tightness by the resistance of the muscle
or the lack of range of motion. The influence of
tightness of the "upper" abdominal muscles in de-
pressing the chest should not be overlooked in this
test.

CHAPTER V

TESTS FOR MUSCLE STRENGTH

Muscle strength testing is a procedure for evaluating the functional strength of muscles. The technique of manual muscle testing* is basically the same in cases of faulty posture as in neuro-muscular conditions but the range of weakness encountered is less and the number of muscle tests that are of practical importance is considerably less.

The authors have repeatedly done complete muscle tests on normal subjects and the results have indicated that certain muscle groups tend to show weakness which is related to typical faults of alignment. These muscles are therefore included in the series of tests which may be regarded as the "minimum essential tests" in a postural examination, and are the muscles listed on the postural examination chart.

Muscle testing is important not only in determining which muscles are weak and in need of strengthening exercises, but also in determining the need for supportive measures. When mild muscle weakness exists along with faults of alignment the individual may respond to a program of therapeutic exercise without supportive treatment. When the muscle weakness is moderate or marked the degree of weakness is an indication of the amount of support needed, and re-evaluation of strength from time to time serves to indicate when use of supports may be discontinued. Muscle weakness may appear secondary to alignment faults or alignment faults may appear secondary to weakness. In the latter case, by making it possible to detect muscle weakness before alignment faults have become habitual or structural, muscle testing serves as a valuable aid in prevention of postural faults.

The specific function of each muscle is determined by the line of pull of its fibers. No two muscles in the body have exactly the same line

* A comprehensive discussion of muscle testing may be found in Muscles, Testing and Function by H. O. and F. P. Kendall, The Williams & Wilkins Co., Baltimore, 1949.

of pull. Thus whenever muscle weakness exists the performance of some exact movement is affected or the stability of some part of the body is impaired.

A muscle test is designed to "isolate" as far as possible the specific action of the muscle to be tested. A test position is a position in which a part of the body is placed by the examiner and held, if possible, by the subject. A test movement is a movement of a part through a specified arc of motion and in a specified direction. In general, for tests of muscles which move the extremities, the subject is asked to hold the part in a specified test position against the pull of gravity and against maximum pressure exerted by the examiner. In the case of finger or toe muscles, however, the weight of the part is negligible and the effect of gravity can be largely disregarded.

A muscle which maintains its anti-gravity test position against this maximum pressure is graded 100 per cent. In many cases 100 per cent strength represents the ability of the muscle to hold the part against sufficient pressure to displace the body weight proximal to the tested part.

If the muscle holds an anti-gravity test position against medium pressure its grade is 80 per cent to 90 per cent; if it holds against minimum pressure its grade is 60 per cent to 70 per cent. A 50 per cent grade means that the anti-gravity test position can be held if no added pressure is exerted by the examiner. This is the most objective grade because the pull of gravity is a constant factor. Because muscle weakness which grades less than 50 per cent is seldom encountered in cases of faulty posture, details about such grading are omitted and it is suggested that evaluation of muscles with less than 50 per cent strength be recorded as "weak". (It is only when the word "weak" is used formally as a test grade that it is used with this limited meaning.)

In the case of anterior trunk muscles, the weight of the part is so great in proportion to the power of the muscles that the pull of gravity alone is sufficient resistance and no additional pressure is exerted by the examiner. Detailed instructions for grading the trunk muscles are included in the descriptions of the tests.

To insure accurate testing the examiner must not permit substitution through assistance given to the muscle being tested by other muscles which have a similar action. This can be prevented by careful adherence to exact test position or test movement, and by applying pressure in direct opposition to the line of pull of the muscle.

Pressure must be applied very gradually in muscle testing. Even a very strong muscle will yield if pressure is applied suddenly.

Tightness of opposing muscles or of joint structures may restrict movement and so limit the range that the part cannot be placed in test position or move through the arc of motion. In such cases grading is based on performance through the existing range rather than through normal range of motion, and grades are recorded in parentheses to indicate that restriction of the arc of motion is present.

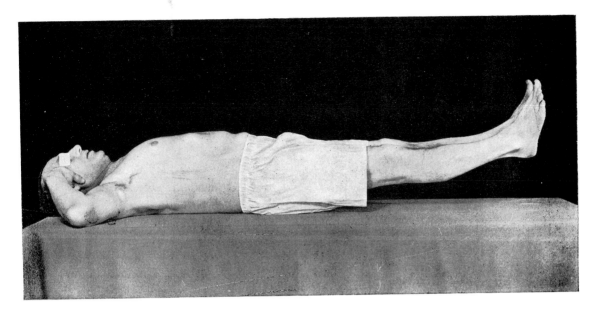

FIG. 100. Leg-raising Test for "Lower" Abdominal Muscles

A person with 100% "lower" abdominal muscles is able to maintain the pelvis in a position of posterior tilt with the back flat while raising both legs from the table. The figure above illustrates the beginning stage of the movement. At this stage the weight of the legs is exerting a maximum pull downward on the pelvis to resist the upward pull on the pelvis by abdominal muscles. (The rectus abdominis and obliquus externus are chiefly responsible for the pelvic fixation during this movement.) The narrowing of the costal angle indicates that the obliquus externus is contracting.

If the subject is unable to initiate leg-raising without allowing the back to arch, the legs are brought (with assistance) to a nearly vertical position and the subject is asked to hold the back flat while slowly lowering the legs. The angle between the legs and the table when the back just begins to arch off the table is used to determine the muscle strength grade. If the angle is about 80° the grade is 50%; if about 60° the grade is 60%; if about 40° the grade is 80%. (Fig. 114 shows the arching of the back due to failure of the abdominal muscles to stabilize the pelvis during a leg-raising test.)

When the "lower" abdominal test is given to patients with back pain an effort is made to avoid strain on the back. The attempt to do double leg-raising is omitted, and the test is done by checking for pelvic tilt during leg-lowering as described above. Also in such cases, the arms are usually crossed on the chest instead of placed under the head as illustrated.

It will be noted that the rectus abdominis is being mentioned as one of the muscles primarily concerned in both the "upper" and "lower" abdominal tests. This does not mean that the action is confined to the upper and lower halves of the rectus respectively. The terms "upper" and "lower" refer not to location of the muscles, but to the section of the trunk which is chiefly involved in the movement. For a more complete analysis of double leg-raising see pp. 50 and 53.

The 100% standard for lower abdominal muscles is primarily a standard for adult males. For other individuals normal strength according to age may be considered as follows: Infants, test not used; age 4–12, 60% to 70%; age 12 to adults, 70% to 80%; adult women, 80%.

The tests for strength of "upper" and "lower" abdominal muscles are important in all routine postural examinations.

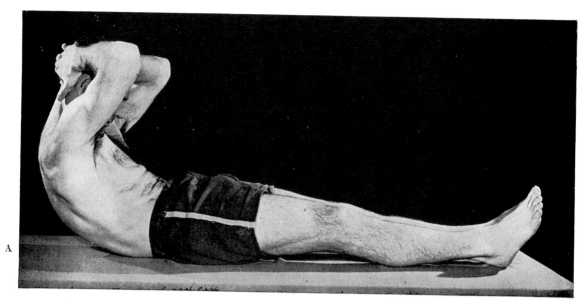

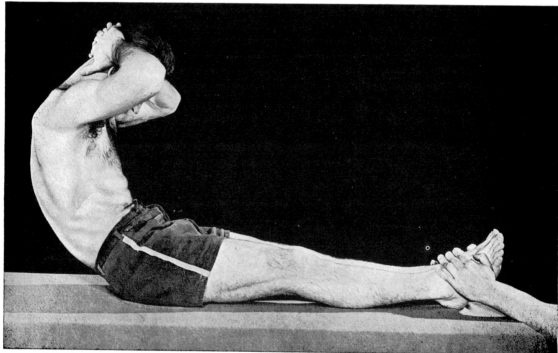

FIG. 101. Trunk-raising Test for "Upper" Abdominal Muscles

This figure shows two stages in the movement used to test the "upper" abdominal muscles. The starting position is supine with the hands clasped behind the head and the pelvis tilted backward to flatten the low back against the table.

Figure A shows flexion of the trunk completed (primarily by the action of the rectus abdominis and the obliquus internus). The subject should come to this position without jerking, raising first his head and then his shoulders. Through this arc, his feet should not come up from the table, but neither should they be held down by an assistant.

The change in the costal angle as abdominal test movements are done indicates which of the oblique muscles is acting. In this test the increase of the angle indicates that the internal oblique muscles are acting because the ribs flare outward.

In B the primary movement is flexion of the trunk on the thighs by the hip flexors. (The obliquus externus joins the internus and rectus in completing and maintaining flexion of the trunk.)

In the second stage of the movement the legs may be held down by an assistant if the weight of the legs does not counterbalance the weight of the trunk.

The arms, as illustrated, are in a position for a 100% trunk-raising test. A grade of 80% is given if the movement can be completed with the arms folded across the chest. In the 60% test the arms are extended diagonally forward during the movement. For the 50% test the same arm position is used as for the 60% test but the 7th cervical vertebra is lifted only about 4 to 5 inches above the table.

If the subject who has normal flexibility of his back is unable to perform the 50% test the muscles are graded "weak". If the back muscles are very tight it must be determined whether abdominal weakness or back tightness has prevented completion of the test movement. For further analysis of the trunk-raising movement see pp. 51 and 53.

Grades for different age levels which may be considered normal in the trunk-raising test for "upper" abdominals are as follows: Infants and very young children, test not used; age 4–5, 40% to 60%; age 6–8, 60% to 80%; age 9–12, 80% to 100%; over 12 years, 100%.

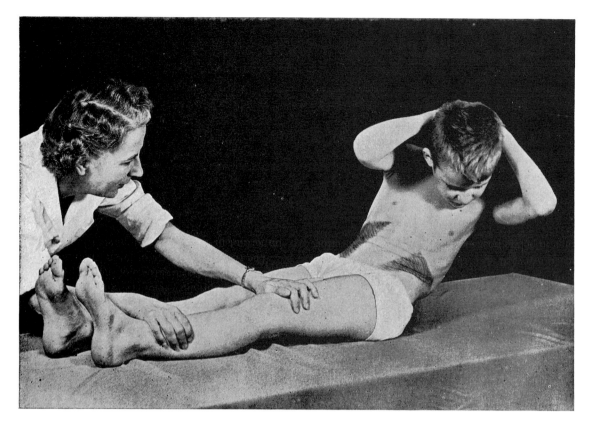

FIG. 102. Trunk-raising Test for Oblique Abdominal Muscles

The figure shows the position for the 100% oblique trunk-raising test. The examiner places the trunk in the exact test position of flexion and rotation and asks the subject to hold that position. If the strength of the muscles is 100% the trunk will not drop or shift out of position. When the trunk is rotated forward on the right, as illustrated, the diagonal fibers of the right external and left internal oblique muscles are chiefly used. If the left side is rotated forward the left external and right internal oblique muscles are used.

The legs must be stabilized by an assistant during the performance of this test, and hip flexor strength must be adequate to stabilize the pelvis in this test position. For an 80% test the arms are folded on the chest and the shoulder is held only a few inches above the table. For a 60% test the arms are extended forward and the lower shoulder is barely lifted from the table. The 50% test does not involve raising the trunk. With the examiner giving moderate resistance against a diagonally downward pull of the subject's arm, the cross-sectional pull of the oblique abdominal muscles should be very firm on palpation and should pull the costal margin toward the opposite iliac crest. The test may also be done by applying pressure against the thigh with the leg in about 60 degrees hip flexion. The obliques should then pull the iliac crest toward the opposite costal margin.

The test of the oblique abdominal muscles is most important in cases of scoliosis.

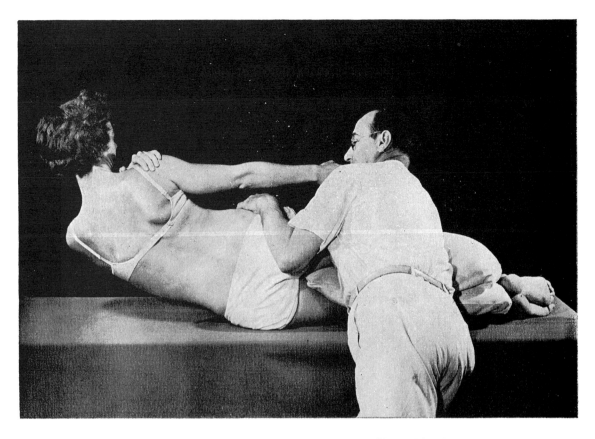

FIG. 103. Test Movement for Lateral Trunk Flexor Muscles

The position shown is the final stage of trunk-raising sideways. The movement starts with the patient lying on his side. The upper arm is held along the side of his body. (The fingers are closed in a fist to keep the subject from assisting by pulling with the hand on the thigh.) The lower arm is folded across the chest and the hand rests on the upper shoulder. As illustrated, pillows are placed on top of and between the legs to prevent the discomfort of one leg pressing on the other. The subject raises the trunk by lifting first the head and then the shoulders sideways. There should be no rotation of the trunk. As the movement progresses, the upper side of the pelvis tilts downward and the upper leg slides downward a little to accommodate for the change in pelvic position. The examiner, in his effort to stabilize the legs, must not prevent this adjustment.

The ability to do this test movement correctly depends upon having a full range of motion in lateral trunk flexion as well as upon having adequate strength.

The lateral trunk flexors are graded 100% if the costal margin can be brought close to the iliac crest. If the lower shoulder is raised about 4 inches from the table the muscle grade is 80%. If the shoulder is raised only 1–3 inches from the table the grade is 50%–60%. If the trunk fails to move through the full arc of motion the examiner must determine whether the primary reason is weakness of the muscles being tested or tightness of their opponents.

The tests for strength of lateral trunk flexors are important in cases of lateral pelvic tilt and scoliosis.

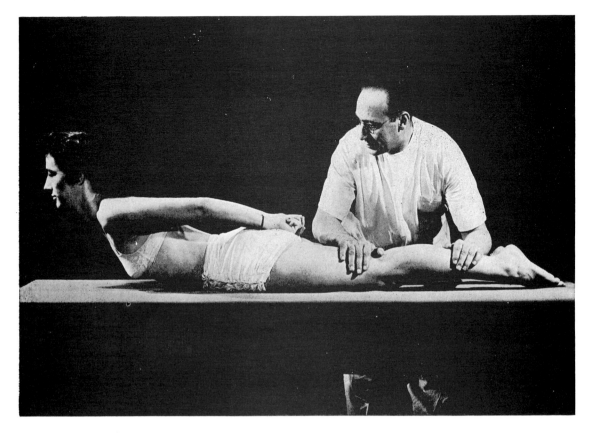

FIG. 104. Test for Back Extensor Muscles

The back extension movement is done as illustrated. If the subject can hold this position against maximum pressure exerted downward on the upper dorsal spine by the examiner, the grade is 100%. If the position is held against slight pressure the grade is 80%. If the subject almost completes the full movement the grade is 60%. If he raises high enough to lift the lower end of the sternum from the table the grade is 50%.

While exerting pressure on the upper back with one hand for the 100% and 80% tests, the examiner continues to stabilize the lower legs with the other hand.

The low back extensors are seldom weak in cases of typical faulty posture. However, since the erector spinae muscles are the most important of all the trunk muscles, it is necessary to detect weakness when it exists. For this reason, and because the routine examination of back extensors will dispel the mistaken idea that most painful low backs are "weak" this test is included in the group for postural cases.

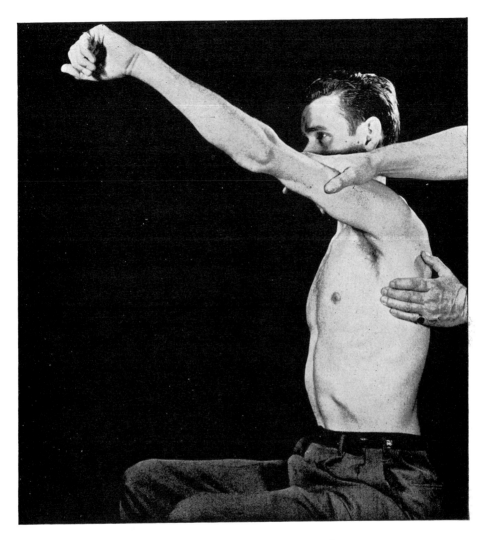

FIG. 105. Test for Serratus Anterior

The serratus anterior holds the scapula close to the rib cage and rotates the inferior angle of the scapula forward. The sitting position illustrated is one of several which may be used for testing this muscle. The arm is placed in about 120° flexion and the subject asked to hold the position while the examiner exerts downward pressure on the upper arm and backward pressure on the scapula. If the serratus anterior is weak the inferior angle of the scapula will rotate medially and the whole vertebral border of the scapula will stand out from the rib cage; the subject will be unable to hold the test position because of lack of adequate scapular stabilization.

Tests for strength of the serratus anterior should be done in cases of faulty scapular position, or in cases of pain in the area of the rhomboids since the latter may shorten and be painful in cases of serratus weakness.

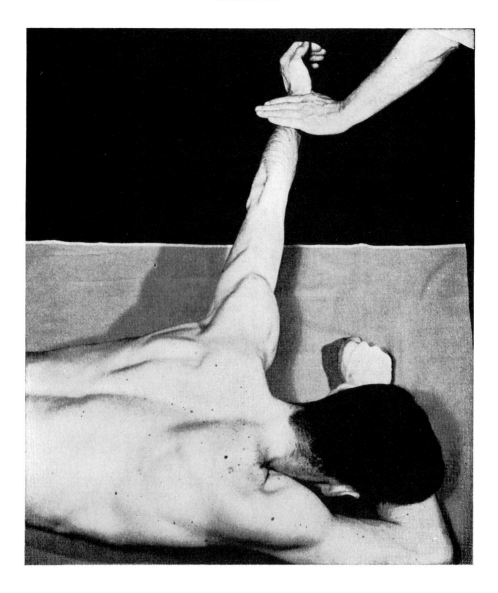

FIG. 106. Test for Middle Trapezius

For this test the subject is in a prone position.

The middle trapezius action in adducting the scapula is best demonstrated when the inferior angle is rotated slightly outward.

This position of the scapula is obtained by placing the extended arm in about 90° abduction and outward rotation and raising it several inches from the table. The subject is asked to hold this position as the examiner exerts downward pressure on the forearm.

The arm cannot be held in the test position unless the scapula is well stabilized in adduction. If the middle trapezius is weak the scapula lacks adequate stabilization.

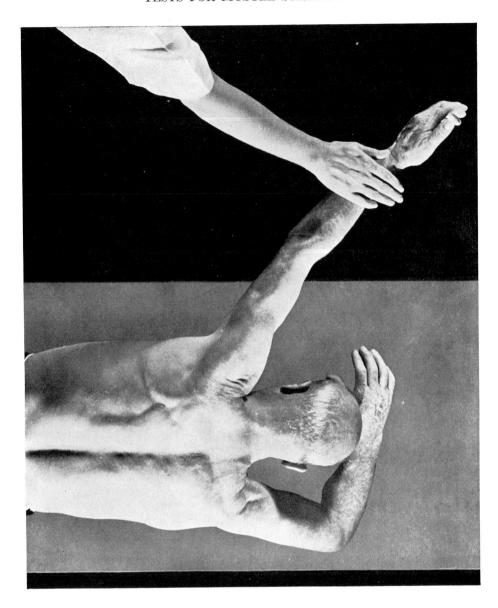

FIG. 107. Test for Lower Trapezius

For this test the subject is in a prone position.

The lower trapezius action in adducting and de-pressing the scapula is best demonstrated when the inferior angle is rotated outward.

This position of the scapula is obtained by placing the extended arm in external rotation in a diagonally overhead position and raising it a few inches from the table. The subject tries to hold this position as the examiner exerts downward pressure on the forearm.

The arm cannot be held in the test position unless the scapula is well stabilized in adduction and de-pression. If the lower trapezius is weak, the scapula lacks adequate stabilization.

Tests for lower and middle trapezius are especially important in examination of cases in which shoulder position is faulty, or in cases of painful upper back or arm conditions.

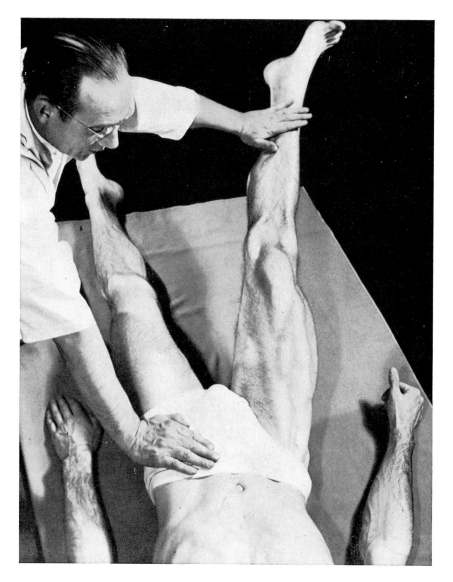

FIG. 108. Test for the Psoas Major

The subject is in a supine position. The examiner places the leg to be tested in a position of hip flexion, slight abduction, and slight external rotation, and asks the subject to hold that position while he presses downward and slightly outward on the lower leg. The examiner stabilizes the opposite hip.

The test for psoas major is of particular importance in cases of anterior deviation of the pelvis, lumbar kyphosis, or lumbar scoliosis. Weakness tends to be bilateral in cases of lumbar kyphosis, and unilateral in cases of lumbar scoliosis.

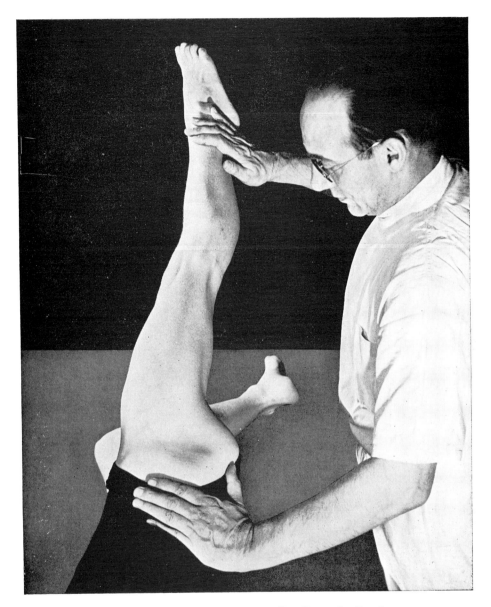

FIG. 109. Test for Gluteus Medius (Posterior Part)

The subject lies on his side with the underneath leg flexed at the hip and knee. The upper leg, which is the one to be tested, is placed in abduction, slight extension, and slight external rotation by the examiner, and the subject is asked to hold this position against pressure. Then the examiner uses one hand to help stabilize the pelvis while with the other he presses downward and slightly forward on the lower part of the leg. Attempts by the subject to substitute by rotating the leg back into a neutral position, by rolling the upper hip backward or forward, or by bringing the thigh into flexion are common. The grade should be determined by the ability to hold against varying degrees of pressure in the designated test position.

Tests for gluteus medius strength are of particular importance in cases of low back pain and in cases of faulty alignment of the lower extremity.

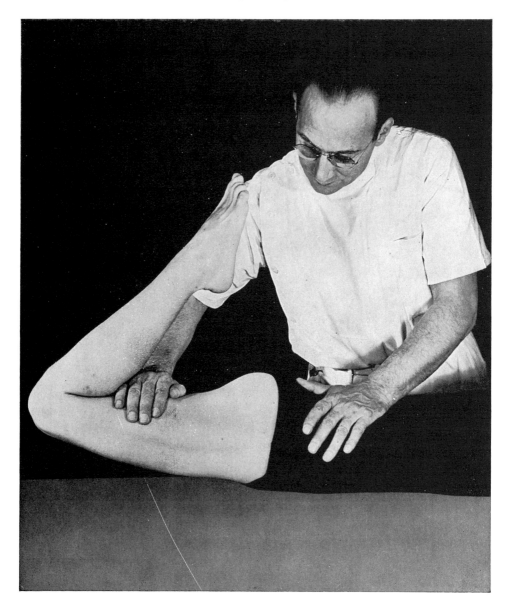

FIG. 110. Test for Gluteus Maximus

For this test the subject is in a prone position. With the knee bent to 90° or more the thigh is raised several inches above the table and the subject is asked to hold this position as downward pressure is exerted by the examiner on the lower part of the posterior thigh.

Testing for strength of the gluteus maximus is of particular importance in cases of anterior pelvic tilt and in cases of coccyalgia. Weakness may be present in the type posture illustrated in fig. 73.

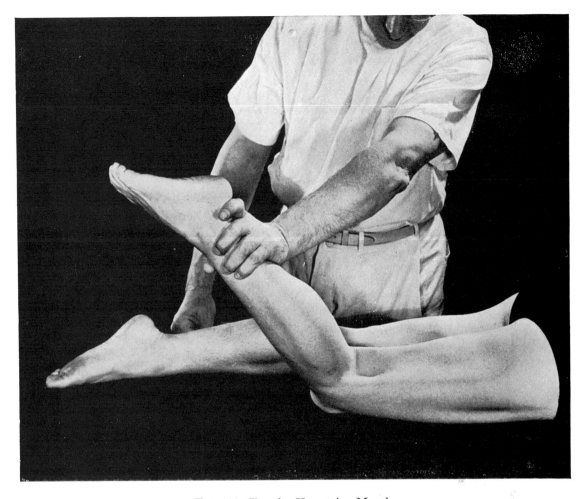

FIG. 111. Test for Hamstring Muscles

With the subject prone, the knee is bent to about a 45° angle. The subject is asked to maintain the position of knee flexion as the examiner exerts downward pressure on the back of the ankle.

Test for strength of hamstrings is of special importance in cases of anterior pelvic tilt and hyperextension of knees.

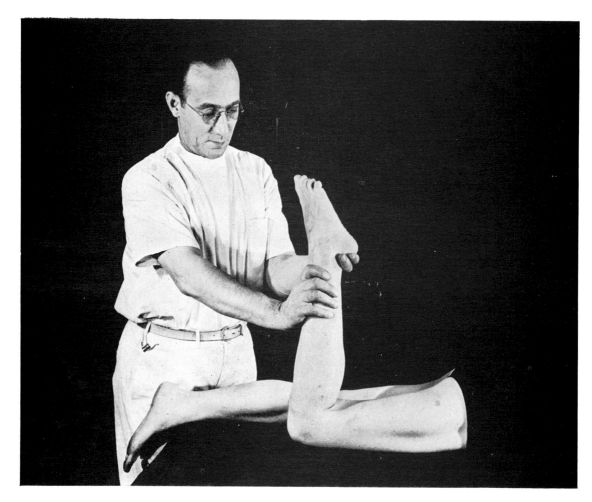

Fig. 112. Test for Soleus

The subject is prone with the knee flexed to at least a 90° angle. The foot is placed in plantar flexion and the subject is asked to hold that position. The examiner provides support for the leg with one hand while with the other he exerts pressure to pull the heel plantarward.

This test is important in examination of cases in which there is a deviation of the body forward from the plumb line. It is also advisable to test this muscle in cases in which there is an increase in the height of the longitudinal arch.

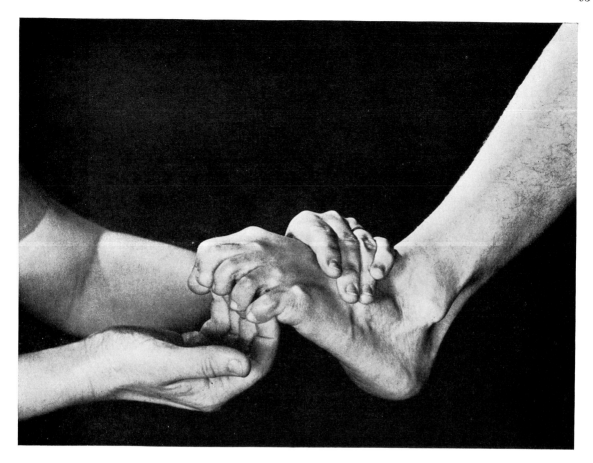

FIG. 113. Tests for Toe Flexor Muscles

The test movement for the flexor hallucis longus is flexion of the distal joint of the big toe. The subject attempts to hold the position as the examiner applies pressure against the distal phalanx.

For the flexor digitorum longus, the subject bends the distal joints of the 2nd, 3rd, 4th and 5th toes and holds against pressure by the examiner.

In pronation of the foot, weakness is frequently found in these two muscles. They are more often weak on the left than on the right because the left foot is generally more pronated than the right.

The flexor brevis is tested by having the subject flex the toes and hold against pressure applied to the middle phalanx.

The test for flexor brevis is important in cases of longitudinal arch strain. A point of acute tenderness is often observed at the place of origin of this muscle on the os calcis.

In the test for flexion by the lumbricales the subject flexes the metatarsal-phalangeal joints of the four outer toes and holds while pressure is applied against the proximal phalanges.

Tests for strength of lumbricales are particularly important in cases of metatarsal arch strain and in cases of hammer toes.

CHAPTER VI
PROCEDURE FOR POSTURAL EXAMINATION

Posture examination consists of three essential parts: 1) examination of the alignment in standing; 2) tests for flexibility and muscle length; and 3) tests for muscle strength.

EQUIPMENT

The equipment used (see fig. 115) consists of the following:

POSTURE BOARDS. These are plywood boards on which foot prints have been drawn. Such foot prints may be painted on the floor of the examining room, but the posture boards have the advantage of being portable.

PLUMB-LINE. The plumb line is suspended from an overhead bar, and the plumb bob is hung in line with the point on the posture board which indicates the standard base point. (See Chapter I.)

FOLDING RULER WITH SPIRIT LEVEL. This is used to measure the difference in level of posterior iliac spines. It may also be used to detect any differences in shoulder level. A background with squares (as shown in many of the photographs in Chapter II) is a more practical aid in detecting differences in shoulder level.

SET OF SIX BLOCKS, 4″ x 10″ of the following thicknesses: $\frac{1}{8}$″, $\frac{1}{4}$″, $\frac{3}{8}$″, $\frac{1}{2}$″, $\frac{7}{8}$″, 1″. These are used for the purpose of determining the amount of lift needed to level the pelvis laterally. This means is preferred to the use of leg length measurement for this purpose (see discussion p. 97).

FLESH PENCIL. The pencil is used for marking the spinous processes in order to observe the position of the spine in cases of lateral deviation.

TAPE MEASURE. This may be used in taking leg measurements, and for measuring the limitation of forward bending in reaching finger tips toward toes.

CHART FOR RECORDING EXAMINATION FINDINGS. (See p. 99.)

APPROPRIATE CLOTHING such as a two-piece bathing suit for girls or trunks for boys should be worn by subjects for a postural examination. Postural examination of school children is unsatisfactory when attempts are made to examine children clothed in the ordinary gym suits.

In hospital clinics, gowns or other suitable garb should be provided.

ALIGNMENT IN STANDING

The subject stands on the posture boards with his feet in the position indicated by the foot prints.

Anterior View

Observe the position of the feet, knees, and legs. Toe positions, appearance of the longitudinal arch, alignment in regard to pronation or supination of the foot, rotation of the femur as indicated by the position of the patella, knock-knees, or bow-legs should all be noted. Any rotation of the head, or abnormal appearance of the ribs should also be noted. Findings are recorded on the chart under "Segmental Alignment".

Lateral View

The relationship of the body as a whole to the plumb-line is noted and recorded under "Plumb-Line Tests". It should be observed from both right and left sides for the purpose of detecting rotation faults. Such descriptions as the following may be used in recording findings: "Body anterior from ankles up", "pelvis and head anterior", "good except lordosis", "upper trunk and head posterior".

Segmental alignment faults may be noted with or without the plumb-line. Observe whether the knees are in good alignment, hyperextended, or flexed; note the position of the pelvis as seen from side view; whether the antero-posterior curves of the spine are normal or exaggerated; head position, forward or tilted up or down; chest position, whether normal, depressed, or elevated; and the contour of the abdominal wall.

Findings are recorded on the chart under "Segmental Alignment".

Posterior View

The relationship of the body or parts of the body to the plumb-line are expressed as good, or as deviations toward the right or left, and are so recorded on the chart. From the standpoint of segmental alignment, one should observe the feet noting the alignment of the tendo-Achillis, postural adduction or abduction of the legs, relative height of the posterior iliac spines, lateral pelvic tilt, lateral deviations of the spine, position of the shoulders and of the scapulae. Rotation of the spine or thorax may be observed with the patient bending forward. Findings are recorded under "Segmental Alignment".

TESTS FOR FLEXIBILITY AND MUSCLE LENGTH

In this group of tests are included the tests for muscle length as described in Chapter IV. Findings are recorded on the chart in the space provided. Forward bending is recorded as "Normal", "Limited", or "Normal +" with the number of inches of deviation from or beyond the toes recorded. On the chart, "Bk" indicates back, "H.S.", hamstrings, and "G.S.", gastrocsoleus. An "X" is used to indicate which of these muscles is tight in case of limitation. (See fig. 151 regarding normal for various ages in this test.)

Forward bending may be checked in the standing as well as sitting position, but the authors consider the test in sitting as the more indicative of flexibility. If flexibility is normal in sitting and limited in standing there is usually some rotation or lateral tilt of the pelvis resulting in rotation of the lumbar spine, which in turn restricts the flexion in the standing position.

Findings in regard to the arm over-head extension tests are recorded as normal or limited, and, if limited, as slight, moderate or marked. Hip flexor and tensor fascia lata tightness are described in like manner.

Trunk extension is the movement of backward bending, and is done in the standing posi-

tion to differentiate the flexibility test of the back from the strength test of back muscles (as done in the prone position). Normally the back should arch in the lumbar region. If hyperextension is limited, the patient may try to simulate the backward bending by flexing his knees and leaning backward. Knees should be kept straight during the test.

Lateral flexion movements are used to test for lateral flexibility of the trunk. The length of the left lateral trunk muscles permits range of motion for trunk-bending toward the right, and vice versa. In other words, if flexibility of the trunk toward the right is limited it should be interpreted as some muscle tightness of the left lateral trunk muscles unless, of course, there is the element of limited spinal motion due to ligamentous or joint tightness.

Among other things, the variation among individuals in length of torso and in space between the ribs and iliac crest make for differences in flexibility. It is impractical to try to measure the degree of lateral flexion. Range of motion is considered to be normal for the individual when the rib cage and iliac crest are closely approximated in side bending.

MUSCLE STRENGTH TESTS

Muscle tests essential in postural examinations are described in Chapter V. They include tests of the "upper", "lower", and oblique abdominals, lateral trunk flexors, back extensors, middle and lower trapezius, serratus anterior, gluteus medius, gluteus maximus, hamstrings, hip flexors, soleus, and toe flexors.

In problems of antero-posterior deviations in postural alignment it is especially important to test the abdominal muscles, back muscles, the hip flexors and extensors, and the soleus. In problems of lateral deviation of the spine or lateral tilt of the pelvis it is especially important to test the oblique abdominal muscles, lateral trunk flexors, and the gluteus medius.

Lateral and antero-posterior deviations of alignment are frequently found in combination, and most of the above tests are then indicated as a part of the examination.

Leg Length Measurements

So-called "actual leg length" is a measurement of length from the anterior-superior spine of the ilium to the medial malleolus. Obviously such a measurement is not an absolutely accurate determination of leg length because the points of measurement are from a landmark on the pelvis to one on the leg. Since it is impossible to palpate a point on the femur under the anterior superior spine, it is necessary to use the landmark on the pelvis. It becomes necessary, therefore, to fix the alignment of the pelvis in relation to the trunk and legs before taking measurements to insure the same relationship of both extremities to the pelvis. Pelvic rotation or lateral tilt will change the relationship of the pelvis to the extremities enough to make a considerable difference in measurement. To obtain as much accuracy as possible, the patient lies supine on a table with trunk, pelvis, and legs in straight alignment and legs close together. The distance from the anterior superior spine to the umbilicus is measured on right and left to check against lateral pelvic tilt or rotation. If there is a difference in measurements, the pelvis is leveled and any rotation corrected so far as possible before leg length measurements are taken.

"Apparent leg length" is a measurement from the umbilicus to the medial malleolus. This type of measurement is more often a source of confusion than an aid in determining differences in length for the purpose of applying a lift to correct pelvic tilt. The confusion arises from the apparent reversal of the picture between standing and lying, which occurs when the pelvic tilt is due to muscle imbalance rather than actual leg length difference. In standing a weakness of the right gluteus medius allows the pelvis to deviate toward the right and ride slightly upward giving the appearance of a *longer* right leg. If the postural fault has been of long standing there is usually an associated imbalance in the lateral trunk muscles in which the right laterals are stronger than the left.

In standing, a fault in alignment will result from the lack of support of a weak muscle which should support the lower extremity or pelvis; in lying, a fault in alignment will more often result from the pull of a strong muscle. In the supine position an individual who has the type of imbalance described above, (i.e., a weak right medius and strong right laterals) will tend to lie with the pelvis higher on the right, pulled up by the stronger lateral abdominal muscles. This position in turn draws the right leg up so that it appears *shorter* than the left.

It is recommended that the need for an elevation on a shoe be determined by measurements in the standing rather than lying position. The boards of various thicknesses (see fig. 115) are used for this purpose.

Interpretation of Test Findings

In the usual case of faulty posture the pattern of faulty body mechanics as determined by the alignment test will be confirmed by the muscle tests if both procedures have been accurate. There may be at times, however, an apparent discrepancy in test findings. The inconsistency may be based on such things as the following: the effects of an old injury or disease may have altered the alignment pattern particularly as related to handedness patterns; effects of a recent illness or injury may have been superimposed on an established pattern of imbalance; a child with a lateral curve of the spine may be in a transition stage between a C-curve and an S-curve.

Except in flexible children, the postural faults seen at the time of examination will usually correspond with the habitual faults of the individual. With children it is necessary and advisable to do repeated tests of alignment, and to obtain information regarding the habitual posture from the parent and teacher who sees them frequently. It is also advisable to keep photographic records of children's posture for a really worthwhile evaluation of postural changes in growing children.

It is of particular importance that girls between the ages of ten and fourteen have periodic examination of the spine because more spinal curvatures occur in girls than in boys, and they usually make their appearance between these ages.

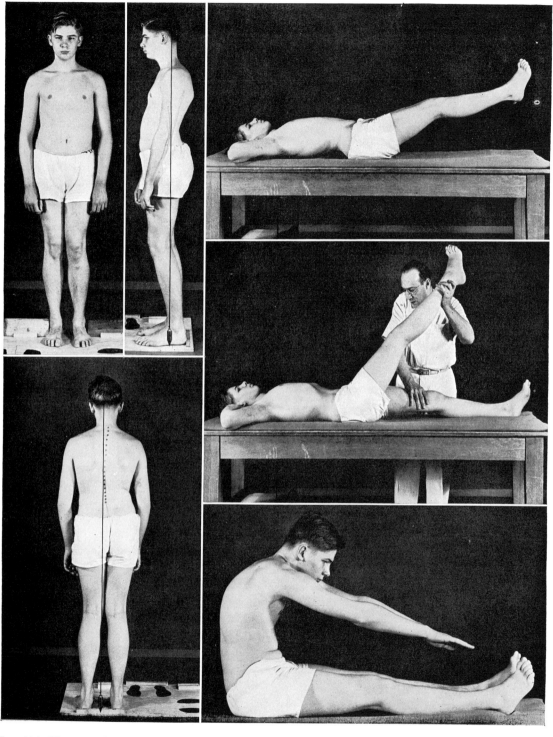

FIG. 114. Photographs showing faulty alignment, limitation of motion in flexibility tests, and abdominal muscle weakness. Examination findings on this case are recorded on the Postural Examination Chart on the opposite page.

CHILDREN'S HOSPITAL SCHOOL
POSTURAL EXAMINATION CHART

Name _D. L._   Date _Feb. 4, 1950_

Diagnosis _Faulty Posture_

Onset _____   Age _17_   Sex _Male_

Occupation _H.S. Student_   Height _____   Weight _____

Handedness _Right_   Leg Length: Left _____ Right _____

PLUMB ALIGNMENT

Side View: From Lt. _Knee, pelvis, & head ant._   From Rt. _(Same as from left)_

Back View: Deviated Lt. _____   Deviated Rt. _Body from feet upward._

SEGMENTAL ALIGNMENT

	X	Hammer Toes		Hallux Valgus			Low Ant. Arch		Ant. Foot Varus
Feet	L.	Pronated >		Supinated			Flat Long. Arch		Pigeon Toes
	B.	Int. Rot. R. > L.		Ext. Rot.	B		Knock-Knees Sl.		Tibial Torsion
Knees		Hyperext. >	B.	Flexed L > R.			Bow-Legs		Deviation
Pelvis	R.	Leg in Postural Add.		Rotation	Ant		Tilt	Ant.	Operation
Low Back	X	Lordosis marked		Flat			Kyphosis		Scap. Elevated
Up. Back	X	Kyphosis		Flat	B		Scap. Abducted R>L	P	Deviation Sl.
Thorax	X	Depressed Chest		Elevated Chest			Rotation	Post.	Cervical -Dorsal
Spine		Total Curve	L.	Lumbar -Dorsal			Dorsal	R.	
Abdomen	X	Protruding Sl.		Scars					
Shoulder		Low		High	B.		Forward	B.	Int. Rotated
Head	X	Forward		Torticollis					

TESTS FOR FLEXIBILITY AND MUSCLE LENGTH

Limited 7"

Forward Bending: Bk. (D-L) Tight. H.S. Tight G.S. Sl. Tight

Arm Over-Head Extension: Lt. Sl. Tight Rt. Normal

Hip Flexors: Lt. Marked Tightness Rt. Marked Tightness

Tensor Fas. Lata.: Lt. Sl. Tightness Rt. Normal

Trunk Extension: Normal

Trunk Lat. Flex.: To Lt. Sl. Limited To Rt. Normal

MUSCLE STRENGTH TESTS

L		R
70	Mid. Trapezius	70
(60)	Low. Trapezius	60
N	Back Extensors	N
100	Glut. Medius	70
N	Glut. Maximus	N
N+	Hamstrings	N+
N+	Hip Flexors	N+
80	Tib. Posticus	100
Weak Lumb.	Toe Flexors	Weak Lumb.

R 90% TRUNK RAISING L
100% Sl. weakness 90%
55% LEG RAISING

SHOE CORRECTION

Left		Right
1/8"	(Wide Heel) Inner Wedge (Narrow Heel)	
3/16"	Level Heel Raise	
Med. Meta. Bar	Metatarsal Support	Med. Meta. Bar
	Longitudinal Support	

TREATMENT

Massage to _____

Infra-red to _____

Diathermy to _____

Exercises:

F. L.:   Pelvic Tilt

B. L.:   Pel. Tilt and Breath.   X

     Pel. Tilt and Leg Sl.   X

     Head and Sh. Raising

     Pectoral Stretch   X

     Hip Flex. Stretch   X

Sd. L.:   Stretch Lt. tensor X

Sit.:   Forward Bending

     To Stretch Low Bk.   X

     To Stretch H. S.   X

     Wall-sitting

     Middle Trap.   X

     Lower Trap.   X

St.:   Foot and Knee Ex.   X

     Wall-standing   X

Other exercises _____

Stretching Toe Extensors.

Cross-sect. - L. Ext. to Rt. Int.

Support _____

NOTES:

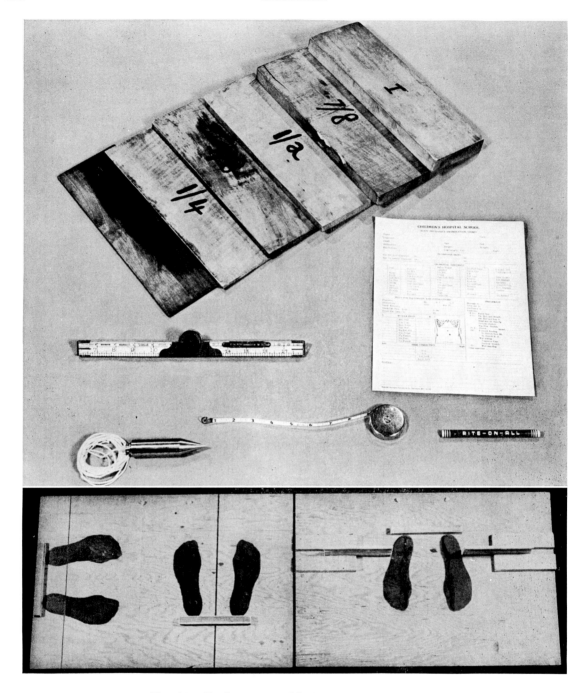

FIG. 115. Equipment Used in Postural Examinations

Set of six blocks, ruler with spirit level, plumb line, tape measure, flesh pencil, chart, and posture boards.

PART III

TREATMENT

CHAPTER VII

PAIN ASSOCIATED WITH FAULTY BODY MECHANICS

A discussion of body mechanics* requires strict adherence to the definition of pertinent terms according to their use in mechanics, except when such is not in accord with recognized medical usage. The terms defined below are essential in the discussion of pain and treatment in relation to faulty body mechanics.

Stress is any force that tends to distort a body. It may be in the direction of either pulling apart or pressing together. Thus skeletal structures (i.e., bones and ligaments) may be subject to stress or they may transmit a stress.

Compression is the force (or stress) that tends to shorten a body or squeeze it together.

Tension is the force (or stress) that tends to lengthen a body or pull it apart. Thus compression and tension are opposite in meaning.

Strain will be used to mean the effect of an injurious tension. This is in accord with medical usage but deviates from the use in mechanics in which strain refers to the force which tends to deform a body or change its dimensions.

Tautness is the result on muscles or ligaments of a non-injurious tension. It implies a state in which slack is taken up to some degree. Because of the elasticity of normal muscle, there exists a range in which tautness is slight, moderate, or marked. In shortened muscles the range is limited and tautness appears before the motion has progressed to the normal limit of joint range. In stretched muscles the part moves to the outer limit of the range of motion before the muscles become very taut. Beyond the point of marked tautness, added tension results in strain.

Stretch means to elongate or extend in length. *Stretch-weakness* is the effect on muscles of remaining in an elongated condition beyond the neutral physiological rest position, but not beyond the normal range of muscle length.

Over-stretch is stretch beyond the normal range afforded by the muscle length.

Shortness or *tightness* are used interchangeably to denote a slight to moderate decrease in muscle length; movement in the direction of elongating the muscle is limited. *Contracture** refers to a marked decrease in muscle length, resulting in an almost complete loss of range of motion in the direction of elongating the muscle. *Irreversible contracture* is one which cannot be released by treatment because elastic tissue has been largely replaced by inelastic tissue.

Throughout this text it is assumed that the role of fascia in relation to the muscle is of basic importance. The related function of muscles and ligaments is also important. The following descriptions from *Gray's Anatomy* (1948 edition) are included to make these relationships self-evident.

LIGAMENTS: "composed mainly of bundles of white fibrous tissue. They are pliant and flexible, so as to allow perfect freedom of movement, but strong, tough, and inextensible, so as not to yield readily to applied force. Some ligaments consist entirely of yellow elastic tissue, as the ligamenta flava which connect together the laminae of adjacent vertebrae. In these cases the elasticity of the ligament is intended to act as a substitute for muscular power."

SUPERFICIAL FASCIA: "found immediately beneath the integument over almost the entire surface of the body. It connects the skin with the deep fascia. . . . Composed of white fibers and yellow elastic fibers."

DEEP FASCIA: "a dense, inelastic, fibrous membrane, forming sheaths for the muscles, and in some cases affording them broad surfaces for attachment. The deep fasciae assist the mus-

---

* The term body mechanics is used in this text with special reference to the skeletal and muscular systems.

* The word contracture is not used here in the same sense that physiologists use it.

cles in their actions, by the degree of tension and pressure they make upon their surface; the degree of tension and pressure is regulated by the associated muscles; as, for instance, by the Tensor fasciae latae and Glutaeus maximus in the thigh, by the Biceps in the upper and lower extremities, and Palmaris longus in the hand."

PAIN MECHANISMS AND TREATMENT INDICATIONS

That faulty body mechanics can cause painful conditions has become a well established concept in the field of Orthopedic Surgery, and is one of the basic concepts in the relatively newer field of Physical Medicine. Such men as Dr. Joel Goldthwaite, who pioneered in the treatment of faulty body mechanics, have laid the firm foundations on which this field of medicine is based.

In discussing pain in relation to postural faults, there are those, however, who are dubious. They often ask the very pertinent question why it is that many cases of faulty posture exist without symptoms of pain. They also question why seemingly mild postural defects give rise to symptoms of mechanical and muscular strain. The answer to both of these questions depends on the constancy of the fault. A posture may appear to be very faulty, yet the individual may be flexible and the position of the body may change readily. A posture may appear to be good but the stiffness or tightness that is present may so limit mobility that position cannot be changed easily. The lack of mobility, which is not apparent as an alignment fault but is observed only in tests for flexibility, may be the more significant fault.

Basic to an understanding of pain in faulty body mechanics is the concept that the accumulative effects of constant or repeated small stresses over a long period of time can give rise to the same difficulties as a sudden severe stress.

Cases of postural pain are extremely variable in the manner of onset, in the severity of symptoms, and in the nature of associated faulty mechanics. There are cases in which only acute symptoms appear, usually as a result of some unusual stress or injury, and in which there is no predisposing faulty body mechanics. Some cases have an acute onset and develop chronically painful symptoms. Some exhibit chronic symptoms which later become acute; others remain chronic.

While immobilization is often a necessary expedient for relief of pain, stiffness of the part is not a desirable end result. The necessity of immobilizing the part is a form of "giving in" to the pain and should be considered a temporary measure except in the event that some serious or irreparable damage has been done that requires continued immobilization. The patient should understand that a transition from the acute stage to recovery requires a change from immobilization to normal motion.

The relief that may accompany immobilization and the fear of repeating the movement which brought on the acute attack may have so impressed a patient that he is reluctant to cooperate in the treatment which aims to increase movement. Recovery depends on cooperation by the patient and this cannot be obtained unless the patient understands the procedure.

Symptoms associated with an acute onset are often widespread and the presence of severe pain makes it impossible to do a detailed analysis of the faulty mechanics. Only after acute symptoms have subsided can tests for underlying faults in alignment and muscle balance be done and specific therapeutic measures be instituted.

The symptoms which are present in the acute stage bear some similarity to the chronic faults. The underlying faults may cause the acute attack, or the distortion of alignment or muscle balance in an acute attack may initiate the chronic faults. The apparent similarities between the acute symptoms and chronic faults should not be construed to mean, however, that the patterns of alignment or muscle reaction are the same but merely more severe in comparing the acute with the chronic. The usual pattern may reverse itself as a compensatory protective means of relieving pain in the acute stage. For example, a patient with acute onset of pain of sciatic distribution in the right leg may stand on his left leg, abduct and externally rotate the right to obtain relief of pain. Seen previous to the acute attack or after the acute symptoms have subsided, he may show the pattern of postural adduction and internal rotation of the right leg in standing.

The table opposite lists the acute symptoms and chronic faults, and the treatment indicated. Each of the topics listed is discussed in detail immediately following the table or along with the section on Exercise.

For an understanding of *pain* associated with the acute symptoms and the faults listed in the table opposite, it is necessary to understand the factors of mechanical stress which give rise to symptoms of pain.

Although it may seem redundant, attention is drawn to the fact that pain—whether it is pain in the muscle, joint, or nerve itself—is a response of the nerve. In other words, regardless of where the stimulus may arise, the sensation of pain is conducted only by nerve fibers. The mechanical factors which give rise to pain must, therefore, directly affect nerve fibers. There are two such factors to be considered in problems of faulty body mechanics:

1. *Tension* on structures containing nerve endings sensitive to deformation as found in stretch or strain of muscles, tendons, or ligaments. The pain may be slight or excruciating depending on the severity of the strain.

2. *Pressure* on nerve root, trunk, nerve branches, or nerve endings caused by some adjacent firm structure such as bone, cartilage, fascia, scar tissue, or taut muscle.

Pain resulting from an enlarged ligamentum flavum or protruded disc exemplifies nerve root pressure.

The "scalenus anticus syndrome" in arm pain and the "piriformis syndrome" in sciatica, described in the literature, are examples of nerve irritation associated with tautness of the respective muscles.

Acute Symptoms and Treatment Indicated	Chronic Faults and Treatment Indicated
1. Muscle spasm Treatment Indicated: Depend on type of spasm.	1. Tightness of muscles and related fascia Treatment Indicated: Heat, massage, and stretching to restore mobility.
2. Strain of muscles or ligaments Treatment Indicated: Immobilization in a position that relieves tension on the affected muscles or ligaments.	2. Stretch-weakness of muscles and ligaments Treatment Indicated: Release of tension by whatever measures are necessary such as: Supports Stretching tight, opposing muscles Followed by: Strengthening exercises for the weak muscles.
3. Undue compression or traction on bone Treatment Indicated: Correction of alignment to relieve bony compression, or to relieve tension imposed by taut ligaments.	3. Faulty alignment Treatment Indicated: Correction of alignment by whatever measures are necessary such as: Supports Restoration of mobility in tight muscles which limit the range. Restoration of strength in weak muscles which fail to maintain alignment.

The distribution of pain along the course of the involved nerve and the areas of cutaneous sensory disturbance are aids in determining the site of lesion. Pain may be localized below the level of direct involvement or may be widespread because of reflex or referred pain. In a root lesion, pain tends to extend from the origin of the nerve to its periphery. The cutaneous sensory involvement is on a dermatome basis. A peripheral nerve involvement is often distinguished by pain below the level of lesion, following the course of the nerve. Cutaneous sensory involvement is on a peripheral sensory supply basis. In cases of muscle strain the pain associated with tension within the muscle may be widespread due to reflex or referred pain mechanisms, or may be outlined by the margins of the muscle. Use of movements which require stretch or contraction of the specific muscle under observation may confirm that the strain is of a particular muscle.

Strain of Muscles or Ligaments

Strain is the effect of an injurious tension. It may result from a prolonged, continuous tension, or from a sudden undue tension. Forces within the body which exert tension on muscles or ligaments are chiefly those arising from a distortion of bony alignment or from some unusual muscle pull. Therefore muscle tension is described in conjunction with muscle spasm, or faults of alignment and mobility.

Muscle Spasm

Treatment of the acute symptoms associated with faulty body mechanics consists chiefly of the treatment of muscle spasm. Such treatment is necessarily based on an understanding of the various mechanisms which give rise to this symptom.

Muscle spasm is an involuntary contraction of muscle or of fibers within a muscle. It occurs as a result of some excessive nerve stimulation. Peripherally it may arise from irritation of the anterior horn cell, nerve root, nerve trunk or plexus, peripheral branches, or nerve endings. The extent of muscles in spasm depends to some degree on the level of the lesion. Irritation from root, plexus, or peripheral nerve branch level will tend to cause spasm of a number of muscles, while spasm due to irritation of the nerve endings within a muscle may be limited to the muscle involved. Pain due to the latter may, however, be widespread due to reflex pain mechanisms.

Muscle spasm may occur secondary to injury of an underlying structure such as ligament, or bone. Such a muscle reaction is labeled a *protective spasm* because it is a way of "splinting" or "immobilizing" the part to avoid movement and further irritation of the underlying structure.

Muscle spasm may occur within a muscle as a result of a muscle injury. Destruction of normal contractility of the injured area allows shortening of the uninjured part which, indeed, may also be stimulated to contract reflexly as a result of the injury. The contraction of this part puts tension on the injured part and a condition of severe strain is present. The involuntary muscle contraction of the uninjured part may be referred to as a *segmental muscle spasm*.

Muscle spasm associated with a tendon injury is similar to the above, but the tension is exerted on the tendon rather than on a part of the muscle. It may be designated as *muscle spasm associated with tendon injury*. In this connection it will be recalled that tendons contain many nerve endings sensitive to stretch, and pain associated with tendon injury tends to be severe.

An involuntary contraction of muscle may occur when a relatively stronger muscle retracts in response to partial or complete loss of the power of contraction by its opponent. For convenience, this may be labeled *muscle-imbalance spasm*.

Secondary to some form of initial nerve stimulation of a muscle, a state of hyperactivity may persist that simulates muscle spasm. The state of contraction of the muscle which results might be secondary to changes in the chemical environment within the muscle resulting, perhaps, in alterations in the contractility of the protein, or actual minute structural damage.

Treatment of muscle spasm depends on the type of spasm. Relief of spasm resulting from *initial nerve irritation* of the root, trunk, or peripheral branch must depend on relief of the nerve irritation causing it. Treatment of the muscle or muscles in spasm will only aggravate the symptoms. For example, one should avoid the use of heat, massage, and stretching of hamstring muscles in cases of acute sciatica. Rigid immobilization of the extremity is also contra-indicated.

Protective muscle spasm should be treated by the application of a "protective support" in order to relieve the muscle of this extraordinary function. Muscle spasm tends to subside rapidly and pain diminishes when a support is applied. As the muscles relax, the support maintains this function of protection to permit healing of whatever underlying injury gave rise to the protective muscle response. Added relief is obtained by the support giving pressure against the muscles in spasm as well as restricting motion of the part. That comfort should come from direct pressure on the muscle may distinguish this type of spasm from that due to initial nerve irritation. In the low back where protective muscle spasm frequently occurs, a brace with a lumbar pad, or a corset with posterior stays bent in to conform to the contour of the low back, may be used for both immobilization and pressure.

In most instances one may assume that the underlying disturbance is severe enough to require the use of a support for at least a matter of days in order to permit healing. On the other hand, it is not uncommon to find, when the acute onset of pain is caused by a sudden exaggeration of movement, that a rigid posture persists because of the fear of movement, rather than because of the continued need for protective reaction. Because there is this possibility, it is often advisable to apply heat and very gentle massage as a diagnostic aid.

Treatment for the segmental-muscle spasm as seen in cases of muscle strain requires immobilization in a position that relieves tension on the affected muscle.

Treatment for the muscle-imbalance type of spasm requires maintenance of the neutral physiological rest position for the purpose of relieving tension on the weaker muscle as well as maintaining a tension on the strong muscle to prevent the occurrence of adaptive shortening.

It may be that chemical alteration as a result of activity is one of the most common causes of painful muscle conditions. Certain muscle conditions which exist without strain or injury suggest this type of basic fault.

In cases of painful faulty body mechanics, such conditions are most frequently seen in the posterior neck, the tensor fascia lata, and in the low back. A feeling of tightness "builds up" in the muscle. It may "creep on slowly" or one may experience an unexpected suddenness of onset.

The stimulation of circulation by the heat, and the mechanical pressure of massage helping to force the flow of blood through a specific part, tend to alleviate the painful symptoms. Treatment reactions are often so dramatic as to appear psychological. The patient suffering from pain in the back of the neck or in the leg along the tract of the tensor fascia lata may be remarkably relieved of symptoms during the course of a single treatment. Occasional occurrence of such symptoms may be an indication of an unusual stress or over-exertion, but the repeated or continuous presence of symptoms in these muscle areas might suggest an underlying chemical or structural disturbance.

Often the residual effects of poliomyelitis in sub-acute and chronic stages provide the extreme in problems of faulty body mechanics both in regard to alignment and muscle balance. Interestingly enough, the acute symptoms of muscle spasm as seen in poliomyelitis are closely allied to those described above. Initial nerve irritation from central or spinal level is the usually accepted basis of spasm in poliomyelitis. However, the muscle-imbalance type of spasm is also very common, as is the segmental-muscle spasm. The latter occurs in poliomyelitis when the disease causes a segmental paralysis within a muscle. Protective muscle spasm, however, probably does not appear in poliomyelitis.

Bone Compression or Irritation Related to Faults in Alignment and Mobility

From a mechanical standpoint, faults in alignment and mobility are of two types, (1) undue compression on articulating surfaces of bone, and (2) undue tension on bones, ligaments, or muscles. Eventually two types of bony changes may occur. Undue compression may result in a "wearing-away" of the articulating surface, while undue traction may result in an increase in bony growth at the point of attachment.

It is a fault in alignment if a deviation is persistent or if it is severe.

It is a fault in mobility if motion is restricted, or if it is excessive.

Persistence of a faulty alignment results in undue compression on the parts of the articulating surfaces which bear constant or repeated stress. The ability to tolerate ordinary stresses decreases as the degree or duration of the fault increases. As a fault in alignment progresses toward the extreme there is added to the factor of undue compression on bony structure the factor of undue tension on ligaments, or by ligaments on bone.

If a postural deviation exceeds the limit of motion permitted by the articulating surfaces it is at once a fault whether it be momentary or persistent. When such a fault occurs it is usually responsible for a sudden onset of acute pain. An abnormal deviation usually is labeled as a slipping, sub-luxation, luxation, or dislocation. These terms, although correctly applied to some faults in alignment, are often inappropriately used.

Lack of mobility is closely associated with persistent faulty alignment as a factor in causing undue compression. When mobility is lost there is stiffness and a certain alignment remains constant. The lack of mobility may be due to restriction of motion by *tight muscles*, or due to the inability of *weak muscles* to move the part through the arc of motion. Muscle tightness is a constant factor tending to maintain the part in faulty alignment regardless of the position of the body. Muscle weakness is a less constant factor because changing the body position can bring about a change in alignment of the part. When there is normal movement in joints, wear and tear on joint surfaces tend to be distributed. If there is limitation of range the wear will take place only on the joint surfaces that represent the "arc of use".

If limitation of range or stiffness occurs with the part in *good alignment* for weight-bearing, there will be a minimum of pain or disability in standing or sitting, but muscle strain may occur on motion. If the part that is restricted by muscle tightness is guarded against any movement that might cause strain, other parts that must compensate for such restriction may suffer the strain instead.

When limitation of motion holds the body in *faulty alignment* the strain and painful symptoms will tend to be constant whether the individual is quiet or in motion.

Excessive joint mobility results in tension on the ligaments which normally limit the range of motion. There is also the factor of undue compression on the margins of the articulating surfaces in cases in which the excessive range is maintained for a prolonged period of time.

Treatment Modalities

Heat, massage, stretching movements, strengthening exercises, and supportive measures are the essential modalities employed in the treatment of faulty body mechanics. Use of the first four modalities applies to the treatment of faulty conditions of muscles, while use of supportive measures applies to the treatment of faulty conditions of muscles, ligaments, bones, and nerves. The discussion following deals with each of these types of treatment.

Heat

The chief purpose for which heat is used in the treatment of painful muscle conditions is to take advantage of its apparent relaxing properties through the stimulation of circulation. Physiologically the mechanism is not clear, but clinically it may be observed that heat has such an effect. It is therefore indicated in the treatment of tight or contracted muscles.

Heat may also be used for its pain-relieving effect. Since pain may be present in either the area of muscle tightness or weakness, there is an obvious temptation to use it in either case. It has been the experience of the authors, however, that if heat is applied to muscles which are weak as a result of strain or fatigue the symptoms of pain usually increase. The heat fails to be therapeutic as a pain-relieving measure because the effect of further relaxation of the muscles increases the imbalance which is the basic problem. Heat applied to tight low back muscles or tight posterior neck muscles is a great aid in relieving pain as well as in facilitating muscle stretch by means of massage and stretching movements. Heat applied to weak upper back muscles usually increases the pain in this region. If the posterior neck or low back is to be treated by use of heat, the upper back is covered to avoid application of heat to that part. A rule that is closely adhered to in the treatment of muscular conditions associated with faulty and painful posture is:

Apply heat to tight muscles

Avoid applying heat to weak muscles

The effectiveness and ease of application of simple forms of heat make them most useful in the treatment of faulty muscle conditions. Heat which gives superficial rather than deep penetration is more often preferable in the experience of the authors. Infra-red lamps, electric pads, or moist heat may be used effectively. Heat should be applied in moderation.

Non-therapeutic effects of heat may accompany over-dosage. An increase of pain should be taken to mean that the type of heat is wrong, or that it is excessive in duration or intensity. Indiscriminate use of heat should be avoided.

Massage

Massage is considered one of the most useful modalities in the treatment of muscular conditions associated with faulty body mechanics. The purposes for which it is used are chiefly to (1) aid in relaxation of muscle through the effect of massage on circulation, and (2) to help stretch tight muscles and fascia through the use of kneading movements.

Massage can be successfully localized to a very small area, or can be applied to a large area. The area of application may be said to be specifically that of the tight muscles being treated. Reaction to over-massage may be seen as exaggerated soreness or even generalized fatigue of the patient, not at the time as much perhaps as on the following day. The length of time of a massage treatment depends both on the size of the area involved and the stage of the painful condition—less being applied in the subacute than in the chronic stage. It is important to avoid the use of massage for muscles which show strain or stretch-weakness.

Exercise

An analysis of indications and contra-indications for exercise requires clear-cut definitions of terms related to this broad subject. Many of the terms used in a discussion of exercise have loose or varied meanings and it is necessary to restrict or qualify their meaning.

Definitions

Of necessity, the word *exercise* will be given two meanings. One is a general usage in which it includes all strengthening exercises and stretching movements as used in *specific* or *therapeutic* exercise procedures. (See definitions below.) These terms modify the word exercise when such use is intended. In all other instances *exercise* refers to a voluntary muscular contraction which produces or helps produce joint motion.* It may occur as a "lengthening contraction" of a muscle, but usually refers to a movement in which the muscle shortens in length.

Movement refers to joint motion in any given direction.

Stretching is muscle lengthening during movement, induced by some force opposing the muscle, but dependent on the gradual relaxation of the muscle being stretched.

Relaxation implies "letting go" or ceasing activity (i.e., ceasing active contraction) by the muscle. (Relaxation of the opposing muscle is a

---

* "Muscle setting" which refers to muscle contraction without joint motion is omitted in the series of definitions relating to exercise.

necessary factor in any exercise movement, and in any stretching movement the muscle being stretched should be relaxed.)

A *passive movement* is one in which there is no voluntary participation by the muscles which would normally perform that movement. Technically the term should be applied only to joint movements in cases of paralysis of associated muscles, or to movement of a part in an unconscious individual. The term is often applied, however, to denote that most or all of the perceptible joint movement is done by another person (or other outside force).

A *specific exercise* is one that is corrective for the fault existing in a specific muscle or muscle group. As such, it is a form of *specific therapy*.

A *therapeutic exercise* is one that is done in such a manner as to be corrective for the faults existing in the individual, and is a *therapeutic procedure*.

The failure to distinguish between these two fundamental differences in exercise therapy results in the paradoxical situation that a so-called therapeutic exercise (specific for a muscle) may be done in such a manner as not to be therapeutic for the individual. For example, a face-lying, dorsal-spine extension exercise is specific for strengthening weak dorsal spine extensor muscles. For a patient with a kyphosis-lordosis posture in whom low back muscles are over-developed, such an exercise is not therapeutic, however, because in the prone position upper back extension cannot be done without also exercising the low back.

Some exercises are neither specific nor therapeutic for the purpose intended. Double-leg-raising from a back-lying position done for the purpose of strengthening weak abdominal muscles is such an exercise. Due to the abdominal weakness the low back arches during this movement and the abdominals are in turn put on a stretch which tends to weaken rather than strengthen them.

Based on the analysis shown in the accompanying chart, the following are definitions of various types of *exercise*, *stretching* and *joint movements*.

Active exercise is an exercise movement in which the muscle produces joint motion without assistance or resistance (other than gravity resistance).

Assisted exercise is an exercise movement in which the muscle is assisted by an outside force which shares in lifting some of the weight of the part. In general use it implies the aid of another person. When intended as other than this meaning it should be modified as follows:

  a. *Self-assisted*—same as above except that the individual himself gives the necessary assistance. (E.g., an individual may use his left arm to assist in exercise movements of the right.)
  b. *Apparatus-assisted*—same as above except that individual is assisted by a mechanical device.
  c. *Gravity-assisted*—only applicable when there is a tight opponent, and a muscle plus gravity pull against it. (E.g., in a marked tightness of the quadriceps an individual may do gravity-assisted hamstring exercise, sitting up with the knee bent as much as gravity and the pull of the hamstring can bend it.)

Resisted exercise is an exercise movement in which the muscle is resisted by an outside force. In general use it implies resistance by another person. When intended as other than this meaning it should be modified as follows:

  a. *Self-resisted*
  b. *Apparatus-resisted*
  c. *Gravity-resisted*—the term may be used specifically to designate such a procedure, but from the practical standpoint it means the same as active exercise.

Resistance is a force used to develop, toward maximum, the potential strength of normal muscle. The amount of resistance that is advantageous for this purpose depends on the capacity and tolerance of the muscle for increased activity. To develop muscle strength to the desired maximum requires the maintenance of a *full load* of resistance but requires at all times the avoidance of excessive or *over-load*. (Load, according to Webster, is the external resistance overcome by a prime mover. Over-load may be defined as in excess of that amount.)

Active stretching is a stretching movement in which the muscle lengthens by the action of its opponent contracting.

Assisted stretching is a stretching movement in which the opposing muscle is assisted by some outside force. In general use this implies the aid of another person. For modification of such meaning the following terms may be used:

 a. *Self-assisted* (stretching)
 b. *Apparatus-assisted* (stretching)
 c. *Gravity-assisted* (stretching)

Forced stretching is a stretching movement in which the resistance of a muscle is overcome by an outside force. In general use it implies force by another person. It is difficult for an individual to do forced stretching for himself because of pain. Mechanical aids may be used for gradual forced stretching. It may be advantageous to do forced stretching with the aid of gravity, but gravity alone cannot do it. This type of stretching should be considered as a last resort because of the inherent danger of tearing the muscle during such movement.

Manipulation is a passive joint movement done (as the word implies) by the hands of another person. It may be gradual or sudden. Usually muscle tightness is present and manipulation involves forced stretching. If done under an anaesthetic, the element of resistance due to pain is eliminated, but one must realize that the degree of tightness observed in the muscles is an established shortness though not necessarily an irreversible contracture. If tightness is severe, one should not expect lasting correction from one manipulation, but should do a series of manipulations to avoid excess muscle tearing with subsequent reactions.

In treatment of acute conditions associated with faulty body mechanics, manipulation is a measure used by some in an effort to correct a distortion of alignment. The rationale of such a procedure is based primarily on the assumption that muscle and ligamentous faults will tend to disappear if alignment is corrected. On the other hand, there are those who treat by immobilization on the assumption that as muscle spasm subsides, normal alignment will be restored. Both approaches fail to meet the needs of the average case suffering from pain associated with faulty body mechanics. Immobilization for the relief of muscle spasm is indicated, but some attention must be given to alignment. Immobilization in a position of faulty alignment may fail to give relief; it may, rather, cause pain to persist.

Gradual stretching may be regarded as *gradual manipulation* and as such is an important form of treatment for conditions of faulty body mechanics. The authors do not, however, recommend *sudden manipulation* for cases of low back pain. They recognize that there are some who successfully treat by this means, and that the secondary symptoms often clear up as suddenly as they appeared when manipulation is successful. The fact that such a procedure is not recommended is not due to a failure to recognize its therapeutic possibilities, but rests on the assumption that it is too difficult, on the basis of existing symptoms, to select the cases which will respond to this procedure. Patients to whom the procedure is mistakenly applied may suffer serious consequences.

The risk of sudden manipulation in acutely painful back conditions probably lies in the danger of subjecting a muscle in spasm to a sudden injurious tension. If a severe muscle strain results, symptoms may be greatly increased and the correction of alignment that was sought by the manipulation may be counteracted by the severity of the alignment fault that occurs secondary to the muscle injury.

SPECIFIC EXERCISE THERAPY

Muscles are capable of contraction and elongation; the quality of elasticity of muscles depends on a combination of these two factors. Exercises are used specifically to strengthen weak muscles, and to lengthen short muscles for the purpose of restoring, as nearly as possible, the elasticity upon which normal muscle function depends.

STRENGTHENING EXERCISES AND STRETCHING MOVEMENTS

Physiological Function of Muscles	Capacity of Muscles	Factor of Assistance or Resistance	Type of Exercise	Who or What Aids or Resists Muscles
Contraction (+)	Capable of full or adequate contraction	Requires no assistance to perform movement (versus gravity)	*Active Exercise*	
	Incapable of complete contraction	Requires assistance	*Assisted Exercise*	(Another Person) or Self Apparatus Gravity
	Capable of forceful contraction	Requires resistance	*Resisted Exercise*	(Another Person) or Self Apparatus Gravity
Stretch (or Elongation) (−)	Capable of relaxation	Requires no assistance other than force of opposing muscles	*Active-Stretching*	
	Capable of partial relaxation	Requires assistance greater than force of opposing muscle	*Assisted-Stretching*	(Another Person) or Self Apparatus Gravity
	Incapable of relaxation	Requires sufficient force to overcome resistance of tight muscle	*Forced-Stretching*	(Another Person) or Apparatus (Gravity may assist the above)

This discussion does not include reference to the involuntary contraction or elongation of muscles which may be associated with neuromuscular disease.

The capacity to contract or elongate may be faulty as a result of persistent use or lack of use as follows:

1. Persistent voluntary contraction results in *hypertrophy* or *over-development*, and, usually, *muscle shortness*.
2. Persistent lack of voluntary contraction results in *disuse atrophy*. (Includes such things as "bed-weakness", or "loss of tone due to inactivity".)
3. Persistent elongation results in *stretch-weakness*.
4. Persistent lack of elongation results in *adaptive muscle shortness*, *contracture*, or, *irreversible contracture*.

Occupational and recreational activities may be regarded as forms of exercise repeated frequently and persisted in for some time. In dealing with faulty body mechanics it is important to be cognizant of the role of these activities and to analyze them in prescribing treatment. When a postural defect appears to be related to occupational or recreational habits the duration or the intensity of the pattern must be altered in some way in order to treat the condition effectively.

Whether adjustment of the occupational factors alone will alleviate the painful symptoms depends primarily on whether the pattern of activity or position has become a fixed pattern in the individual in the form of muscle tightness or weakness. Usually a condition which has reached the painful stage is one in which some muscle imbalance is present, and specific treatment should be given to the individual in the form of heat, massage and stretching movements for the tight muscles.

Stretching movements must be done gradually to avoid damage to tissue structures. Tightness that has occurred over a period of time must be given a reasonable time for correction. A period of several weeks is usually necessary for restoration of mobility in muscles exhibiting moderate tightness.

Treatment of muscle weakness requires consideration of the factors of muscle-stretch and disuse that are the underlying faults. In cases of faulty body mechanics there are numerous instances of muscle-stretch weakness while the element of disuse atrophy is much less common.

To some degree the lack of opportunity to use muscles because of occupational restrictions, the lack of necessity to use them to capacity, or the state of semi-immobilization imposed by tightness of an opposing muscle results in weakness from disuse. This type of weakness is usually superimposed on the same muscles affected by stretch-weakness. The muscles that are most often affected by stretch and disuse weakness are the abdominals, upper back erector spinae, middle and lower trapezius, and anterior vertebral neck flexors.

Stretch-weakness, being the result of persistent tension on the muscle, must be treated by relief of tension. Re-alignment of the part, bringing it into a neutral position, is the essence of this treatment. Use of supportive measures to help restore and maintain such alignment until weak muscles recover strength is a most important factor in treatment. Any opposing tightness which tends to hold the part out of alignment must be corrected in order to relieve tension on weak muscles. Faulty occupational positions which impose continous tension on certain muscles must also be adjusted or corrected.

When the tension on the weak muscle has been relieved, exercises to help restore strength are indicated. Care must be taken not to over-work a muscle which has been subjected to a prolonged tension stress. In practical application, treatment usually begins with the use of three or four movements of contraction, increasing to six or eight by the end of ten days or two weeks. It is seldom advocated that specific exercises be done more than once a day, but as soon as the strain is relieved, and the part capable of good re-alignment, the patient is expected to use the muscles in their normal function of maintaining good alignment. He should know that it is important to try to maintain good align-

TREATMENT
OF
POSTURAL FAULTS

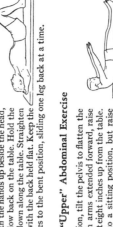

INDIVIDUAL INSTRUCTIONS

The general and specific instructions in this folder are given to help you carry out the necessary follow-up treatment for correction of your postural faults.

The exercises and other treatment selected for you on the basis of your posture examination are indicated on the following pages. An (X) appears in the square beside the paragraph describing the treatment you should do at home.

Heat and massage are used to help relax tight muscles and should precede the stretching exercises. Muscles which are to be stretched should be in a position of slight stretch while the heat and massage are applied.

Exercises in the lying position should be done on a firm table or on the floor. For comfort a thin mattress or folded blanket should be placed on the hard surface.

Strengthening exercises should be done slowly and you should try to get a strong pull by the muscles which are being exercised. The completed position should be held for several seconds before relaxing. The exercises should be repeated the number of times indicated at the back of the folder.

In the stretching exercises, there should be a constant effort to relax the muscles being stretched. The stretching should be gradual, and sufficient to cause mild discomfort. Return the part gradually from the stretched position.

Specific exercises are done to improve muscle balance. To be effective they should be done every day, and continued for a period of weeks until normal length has been restored to the tight muscles, and until the weak muscles have regained their strength. The purpose of the treatment is to restore good posture. This involves the specific treatment outlined to restore muscle balance plus daily practice in assuming a good position until good posture becomes a habit.

While working to correct muscle imbalance associated with faulty posture, it is advisable to avoid certain exercises. Generally the following should be avoided: Lying on the back and raising both legs at the same time; lying on the back and coming up to a sitting position with the feet held firmly down; lying on the back (with most of the weight resting on the upper back) and doing the "bicycling" exercise; from a face-lying position, raising the trunk to arch the back.

Low Back Stretching

In the face-lying position, place a firm pillow under the abdomen and a rolled blanket under the ankles.

□ Have heat and massage applied to the low back while lying in this position. (About...... min. heat and...... min. massage.)

Roll pelvis over the pillow to flatten the low back by pulling down with the buttocks and hamstring muscles.

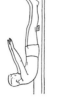

"Lower" Abdominal Exercise

□ In the back-lying position, place a rolled blanket or small pillow under the knees. With the hands up beside the head, tilt the pelvis to flatten the low back on the table by pulling up and in with the lower abdominal muscles. Hold the back flat and breathe in and out easily, relaxing the upper abdominal muscles. (There should be good chest expansion during inspiration, but the back should not arch.)

"Lower" Abdominal Exercise

□ In the back-lying position, bend the knees and place the feet flat on the table. With the hands up beside the head, tilt the pelvis to flatten the low back on the table. Hold the back flat and slide the heels down along the table. Straighten the legs as much as possible with the back held flat. Keep the back flat and return the knees to the bent position, sliding one leg back at a time.

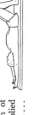

"Upper" Abdominal Exercise

□ In the back-lying position, tilt the pelvis to flatten the low back on the table. With arms extended forward, raise the head and shoulders about eight inches up from the table. (Do not attempt to come to a sitting position, but raise the upper trunk as high as the back will bend.)

Pectoral Self-Stretching

In the back-lying position, bend the knees and place the feet flat on the table.

□ Place the .... arm overhead in a position of slight pectoral stretch, and have heat and massage applied to the pectoral region while in this position. (About...... min. heat and ...... min. massage.)

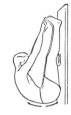

□ With back held flat on the table, extend both arms overhead. Try to touch the entire arm to the table with elbow straight. Bring upper arm as close to the sides of the head as possible.

Low Back Stretching

□ Sit with legs extended forward. Place a rolled blanket under the knees to allow slight knee-bend. Pull in with the abdominal muscles, keep the pelvis tilted back, and reach forward toward the toes, bending the low back. The stretch should be felt in the low back, not under the knees or in the upper back or neck.

Upper Back and Middle Trapezius Exercise

☐ Sit on a stool with the back against a wall. Place the hands up beside the head, and flatten the low back against the wall by pulling up and in with the lower abdominal muscles. Straighten the upper back, press the head back with the chin down and in, and pull the elbows back against the wall.

Upper Back and Lower Trapezius Exercise

☐ Repeat the above exercise. Keep the back and head against the wall. From the elbow-bent position move the arms upward to a diagonally overhead position, keeping the arms in contact with the wall. Occasionally stretch the arms to a straight overhead position.

Foot and Knee Correction

☐ Stand with feet straight ahead and about two inches apart. Relax the knees into an "easy" position, i.e., neither stiff nor bent. Tighten the muscles which lift the arches of the feet, rolling the weight *slightly* toward the outer borders of the feet. Tighten the buttocks muscles to rotate the legs slightly outward (until knee-caps face directly forward).

Standing Postural Exercise

☐ Stand with back against a wall, heels about three inches from the wall. Place hands up beside the head with elbows touching the wall. Correct the feet and knees as in the above exercise. Then tilt the pelvis to flatten the low back against the wall by pulling up and in with the lower abdominal muscles. Repeat the above exercise. From the elbow-bent position move the arms upward to a diagonally overhead position keeping the arms in contact with the wall. Occasionally stretch the arms to a straight overhead position.

Additional Exercises

Use heat and massage...... time(s) daily for the length of time indicated for each treatment.
Start by doing each exercise that has been checked (X)...... times,...... time(s) **daily.**
Increase gradually to...... times, ... time(s) daily by the end of ...... weeks.

Hamstring Stretching

☐ Sitting with knees straight, reach forward toward the toes. Try to bend at the hip joints by tilting the pelvis forward. A stretch should be felt under the knees and along the hamstring muscles.

Hamstring Stretching

☐ In the face-lying position apply heat to the back of the thighs. (About ...... min.)

Place the foot-end of the treatment table against a wall. Lie on the back near the foot-end of the table with the knees bent and feet flat on the table, the toes touching the wall. Move the hips as close to the wall as possible.

☐ To stretch the right hamstrings, straighten the right knee and rest the heel against the wall. Have massage applied to the back of the thigh with the leg in this position. (About ...... min. massage.) To obtain more effective stretch by movement, lie on the table with legs extended and have an assistant hold the left leg down and gradually raise the right with the knee straight.

☐ To stretch the left hamstrings apply the same procedures to the left leg.

Hip Flexor Stretching

☐ To stretch the right hip flexors, lie on the back with the left knee bent (the foot resting on the table), and with the right leg straight. Have heat and massage applied to the front and outer side of the right thigh. (About ...... min. heat and ...... min. massage.) Lie on the back with the right lower leg hanging over the end of the table. Pull the left knee firmly toward the chest to help press the back flat down on the table. (Due to the hip flexor tightness this position will bring the right thigh up from the table.) Keeping the back flat stretch the right hip flexors by pulling the right thigh downward, trying to touch it to the table.

☐ To stretch the left hip flexors, lie with the right knee bent and have the heat, massage and stretching applied to the left thigh as described above for the right.

Tensor Fascia Lata Stretching

☐ To stretch the left tensor lie on the right side with the right hip and knee bent. Relax the left leg on pillows placed between the thighs and lower legs. Have heat and massage applied to the outer side of the left thigh from the hip to the knee. (About ...... min. heat and ...... min. massage.) Remove the pillows. Have an assistant hold the pelvis firmly with one hand, draw the thigh slightly back, and press it downward toward the table stretching the muscles and fascia between **the hip and knee. (The knee should not be allowed to rotate inward, and care should be taken to avoid strain at the knee joint.)

☐ To stretch the right tensor, lie on the left side and have heat, massage, and stretching applied to the right thigh in the same manner as described for the left above.

ment *most of the time*. When a faulty position is assumed more often than a good one, the posture tends to become faulty.

THERAPEUTIC EXERCISE PROCEDURES

The "Treatment Instruction" folder (pp. 114–115) is an outline of various therapeutic measures. It presents brief descriptions (with illustrations) of the physical therapeutic measures of heat, massage, exercises, and stretching movements that are most frequently needed in correction of postural faults. It is given as a guide to patients for the necessary follow-up treatment. The exercises included in this list* are basically the same as have been in use by the authors for the past seventeen years.

Exercises for specific faults are described in connection with the painful conditions discussed in the succeeding chapters.

This book does not include a presentation of therapeutic exercises for scoliosis cases. However, the authors would like to point out that careful muscle examination should be the basis for determining specific and therapeutic exercise procedures in this as in other types of faulty body mechanics. The muscle testing procedures are necessarily more detailed than those outlined in Chapter V of this text.

Muscle testing usually reveals some imbalance in the muscles of rotation of the trunk, particularly in the oblique abdominal muscles. As a rule exercise procedures necessarily include

---

* List first appeared in a private publication entitled "Study and Treatment of Muscle Imbalance in Cases of Low Back and Sciatic Pain" by Henry O. Kendall and Florence P. Kendall, February, 1936. Later reprinted in The Physiotherapy Review, Volume 16, Number 5, September–October, 1936.

exercises to balance the diagonal pull of these muscles. Usually, also, there is lateral pelvic tilt present for which shoe corrections are used as indicated.

Exercises may suffice in cases of mild scoliosis, but in most cases referred for conservative treatment, the combination of supportive measures and exercise are used. The support may be a corset, or a cellulose jacket as in Fig. 124.

Lists of specific exercises, for reference use only, may be made out in order to have adequate and proper wording for description of each exercise. Since specific exercises must be very carefully combined in order that they be therapeutic for each individual case of scoliosis, it is not wise to have any prepared list of scoliosis exercises, but rather a list should be prepared for each individual case.

Since changes of alignment cause changes in the normal patterns of fixation, many otherwise specific exercises have to be adapted in scoliosis work. They also must be changed at various times according to the progress of the individual.

Psoas major weakness is seen quite frequently in cases of lumbar scoliosis. The deviation of the lumbar spine is away from the side of weakness. Psoas major exercise is indicated but it is not advisable to do it in the supine position. Sitting with legs bent over the side of the table and with the back straight or slightly arched, hip flexion, raising the thigh only two or three inches off the table, is done against slight self-resistance. An assistant should observe the back during the exercise to make sure the alignment is corrected in the lumbar region but that it does not deviate into over-correction of the dorsal region.

Mechanical Supports

The mechanical appliances described and illustrated in this section are those specifically used to support the upper and lower trunk. Supports are used for various reasons: (1) to immobilize a part, (2) to correct faulty alignment, (3) to relieve strain on weak muscles, or (4) to restrict movement in a given direction. The legends accompanying the illustrations indicate the chief uses of the various supports. The discussion of muscle weakness (p. 113) explains the basis for use of supports for weak muscles. Correction of alignment faults associated with weakness often requires supportive measures but such measures may not be effective if tightness exists in muscles opposing the weak ones. Application of a support in a faulty position will not relieve strain on the weak muscles. The contracted muscle must be stretched. A support which is adjustable and can help maintain the correction obtained by treatment may facilitate and hasten recovery.

One is often confronted by the specific question, "Should a person with weak abdominal muscles be advised to wear a corset or will he rely on a support to such an extent that the muscles will get weaker if he wears it?" Use of "trial and error" to "feel out the reactions" of the patient in regard to supportive measures may be minimized if muscle testing procedures are employed. The degree of weakness is the most logical basis for determining whether a support is necessary.

Extreme weakness which is due to strain or fatigue will require bed rest or localized rest of the part by the application of a support. Moderate weakness may or may not require support —depending to a great extent on the occupation of the individual. Mild weakness of muscles will usually respond to localized exercise without support or reduction of functional activity. In terms of abdominal muscle strength, in adults any weakness 60 per cent or below is considered in need of support.

Whenever a support has been applied, the question arises, how long will the support be needed? The support will need to be permanent only if the part supported has been irreparably weakened; for example, by paralysis or injury. However, by far the majority of conditions of muscle weakness associated with postural faults can be corrected, and consequently supports need be only temporary until muscle strength has been restored. If no treatment other than the support is used, the individual may become so dependent on the support that it cannot be removed. But if it is understood that therapeutic exercises are to supplement the wearing of the support so that later it may be abandoned, then supports become only an aid to correction rather than a permanent part of treatment.

It is often difficult to convince an individual that wearing a support will help bring about an increase in the strength of his muscles. Such a statement appears contrary to general knowledge that exercise and activity will increase muscle strength. One must explain to the patient that instead of his particular muscle weakness being caused by lack of exercise, it is caused by continuous strain. The support will relieve the postural strain and allow the muscles to function in their normal position.

Bed rest may be indicated for some conditions for the sake of relieving fatigue or muscle strain. It may be used in conjunction with immobilization but should not be considered as a form of specific immobilization for such a condition as a painful low back. The type of mattress is a most important factor when bed rest is indicated. It should be very firm and not sag under the weight of the body. The value of a firm mattress may be lost if the bed-springs permit the mattress to sag. A bed-board placed between the mattress and bed-springs may provide the necessary firmness.

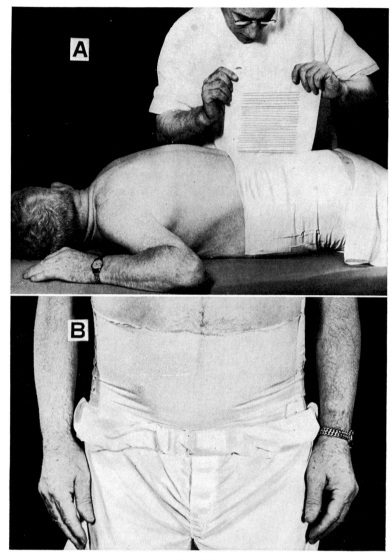

FIG. 116

The above illustrations show an effective back-strapping for acute low back strain. (This type of strapping was first shown to the authors by Dr. Donald Slocum.) As shown in fig. A, a piece of muslin is placed under the abdomen with the patient in a prone position and the adhesive strips are anchored to the muslin on either side. A series of applicators, put on to an additional patch of adhesive, is then placed over the low back.

The applicators are usually broken by gentle pressure so they conform to the low back, and then several additional strips of adhesive applied. The muslin acts to give some abdominal support as shown in fig. B. Wide stockinet may be substituted for the muslin.

This strapping can be used for those needing only temporary support, or used until a more rigid support can be made.

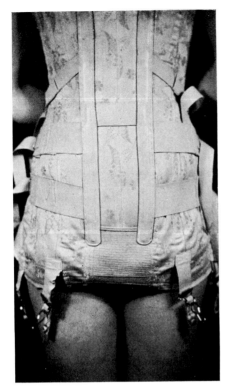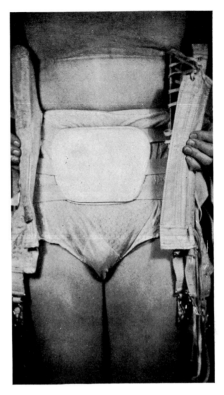

FIG. 117

The above illustration shows a front-lace corset of the type used in some cases of low back pain in which correction of the lordosis plus abdominal support is indicated. A "Goldthwaite" type of support is incorporated into the corset. The steels on the back are about 3½″ apart and are covered with leather.

An abdominal pad which fits inside the corset is attached by means of straps that go through the sides of the garment. In this type of support the steel bars purposely do not conform to the lordotic position, but are practically straight and "bridge" the lordosis, permitting the abdominal pad to lift the abdomen up and back, and thereby to help decrease the lordosis.

The effect of a corset may vary considerably according to the way it is put on. It may merely compress abdominal contents, or it may lift and support them. This is especially true if the abdominal wall tends to be at all pendulous. Organs within the abdominal cavity are displaced downward when in a standing position, but tend to fall back into place in a lying position. If a corset is put on while the individual is lying down, there will be less downward displacement of the abdominal organs when the person stands.

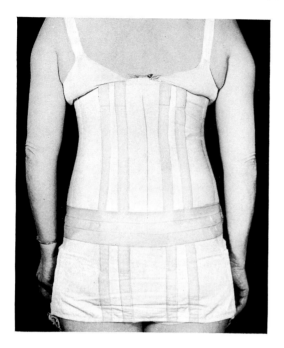

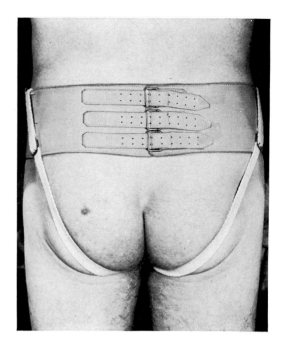

FIG. 118. The corset shown above is a front-lace garment with strong steels at the back and sides. It is fitted to the individual in such a way that it helps transmit the weight of the upper trunk to the pelvis thereby relieving the lumbar spine of some of the weight-bearing. The garment shown above has a sacroiliac strap attached. The corset is made with or without such added support depending on the case.

FIG. 119. The above illustration shows a leather sacro-iliac support with perineal straps to help keep the support in place. The belt is drawn tight around the pelvis to help immobilize the sacro-iliac region.

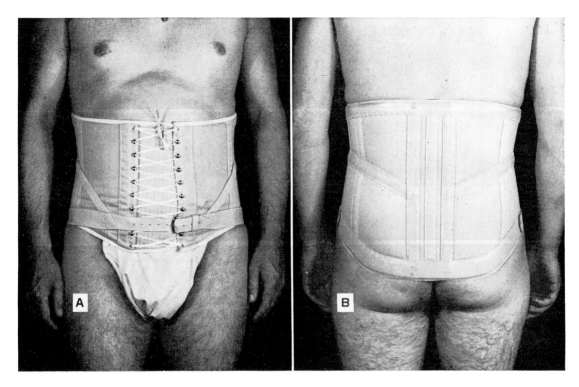

FIG. 120

The above illustrations show the front and back views of a Bennett Back Brace. The steel brace which grips the pelvis and thorax is incorporated in a canvas support.

This type is used more often for men than for women. It is effective not only in relieving weight-bearing on the lumbar spine, but immobilizes the low back against movement in all directions.

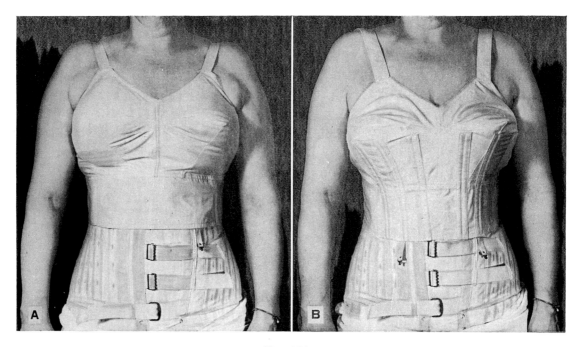

FIG. 121

The figures above show the difference in support obtained by minor changes in a brassiere. Both are exactly the same type of brassiere except that narrower straps are on the brassiere in fig. A and featherbone stays have been added to the one seen in fig. B.

When the weight of heavy breasts is raised and supported by shortening the straps on a brassiere, particularly if the straps are narrow, the pressure is excessive over the shoulders. Such pressure has been observed to be a causative factor in some cases of arm pain. Making straps wider helps distribute pressure but does not relieve it. The addition of featherbone stays which extend upward from the diaphragm-band to the lower half of the cup of the brassiere gives support to the breasts without any shoulder strap pressure.

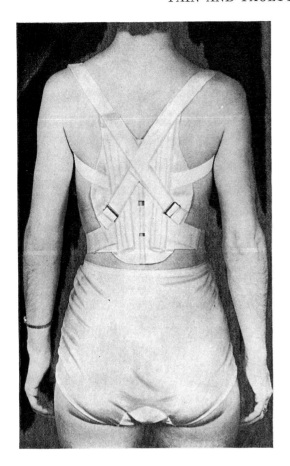 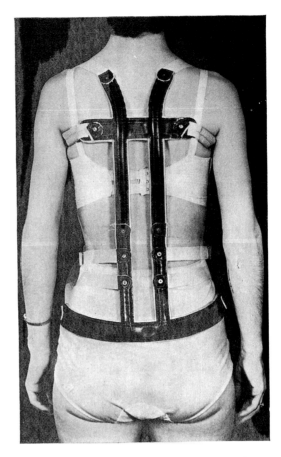

FIG. 122. The shoulder support illustrated above is made of canvas, reinforced with stays. Straps with inserts of elastic loop around the arm in front, cross diagonally over the shoulders in back passing through loops on the support, and are attached by buckles to the lower part of the support. A belt fastens securely around the lower thorax and holds the support in place. This type of support is used extensively in cases of upper back or arm pain associated with faulty shoulder positions.

FIG. 123. The above illustration shows a Taylor Spinal Brace.

In cases of round upper back with or without associated lordosis, it is sometimes necessary to use a rigid support such as this. A pad, similar to that seen in fig. 117, fits over the lower abdomen and is held in place by straps attached to the posterior steels.

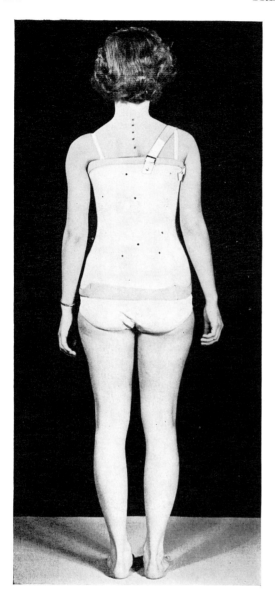

FIG. 124

FIG. 124. Cellulose Acetate Jacket

The patient shown is wearing a removable cellulose jacket of the type used for scoliosis cases. A description of the procedure for making this jacket follows.

The patient is placed in a standing position with head traction from a Sayre head sling. A heel raise to level the pelvis, or strips of adhesive tape put diagonally across the abdomen under the stockinet are used as indicated to obtain the best possible correction of the trunk position before the original plaster cast is applied. For girls, a brassiere with small extra padding is put on under the stockinet in order to allow room for normal development of the breasts.

After the positive plaster mold is poured and is dry, further adjustments may be made by shaving down slightly on the side of convexity and adding an equal amount of plaster at places of concavity at the same level to maintain the circumference measurements necessary.

The cellulose jacket is made by putting four layers of stockinet over the positive plaster mold, and painting each layer of stockinet with four coats of cellulose acetate mixture.* Time should be allowed for each coat to dry before applying the next coat or the next layer of stockinet.

The jacket is cut down the front, removed from the mold and carefully cut to fit the patient. In front it should extend about $\frac{1}{2}''$ below the anterior superior iliac spines. It is finished with leather on the upper and lower borders. It has hooks and lacing down the front. The jacket is made comfortable by padding with thin sponge rubber covered with leather inside the jacket over the iliac crests or other bony prominences. Holes are bored in the jacket for ventilation.

The jacket illustrated has a strap added to help hold the shoulder back.

* Formula for Cellulose Acetate Mixture
Fill a 2 quart jar $\frac{2}{3}$ full of cellulose flakes
Add 3 oz. sizing (Dimethyl Phthalate A)
Fill jar with Acetone U.S.P. XII (C_3H_6O)
Stir as necessary and add acetone as required to keep at about the same consistency as when first dissolved. Use a brush and apply the mixture like paint. (This formula has been used at the Children's Hospital School since 1933.)

CHAPTER VIII

PAINFUL CONDITIONS OF THE LOW BACK, LEG, KNEE, FOOT

The mechanics of the low back is inseparable from the mechanics of the pelvis and lower extremity in relation to posture. Frequently pain manifested in the leg is due to an underlying difficulty in the back. Conversely the symptoms appearing in the back may be due to underlying faulty mechanics in the muscles of the legs and pelvis. Most commonly, however, symptoms and underlying faults appear in the same area.

For careful analysis of any faulty posture problem, examination should not be limited to the area in which the symptoms exist, but should include examination of related parts.

The physical examination findings in regard to symptoms, faulty alignment, and muscle imbalance, and the treatment indications based on these findings, are presented in this chapter.

Low Back Pain

The painful conditions discussed under this category are Lumbo-Sacral Strain, Sacro-Iliac Strain, Facet-Slipping, and Coccyalgia.

Lumbro-Sacral Strain

Lumbo-sacral strain is the most common of the various types of painful low back conditions.

The word strain, used to denote the effect of an injurious tension, does not fully indicate the mechanical faults present in this type of low back pain. There are essentially two problems of mechanics involved. One is the problem of *undue compression* of bony structures, present especially during weight-bearing (i.e., standing or sitting); the other, the problem of *undue tension* on muscles and ligaments, present especially during movement. These may exist in combination or either may be present without the other.

A back may be in good alignment in weight-bearing, but if the posterior muscles are tight, they will be subjected to undue tension in a sudden or "unguarded" attempt to bend forward. Acute pain follows the muscle strain.

A back may have a very faulty alignment, such as a lordosis, without tightness of posterior muscles. Movement then does not cause muscle strain, but standing for any length of time does give rise to pain. The constant stress in the direction of compression, if continued beyond tolerance in time or degree, evokes the painful symptoms. When a combination of faulty alignment and muscle tightness is present, both position and movement may give rise to pain. Pain tends to be constant though it may vary in intensity with change of position. Stresses, which under ordinary circumstances may not have been excessive, may cause a strain. An apparently inconsequential act may cause an acute onset of symptoms.

In cases of low back pain in which alignment is not necessarily faulty, but in which muscle tightness of the back is a major factor, the onset of pain is more often acute than chronic. Pain is increased by, and tends to have its onset in, movement rather than in weight-bearing. It may be relieved by recumbency or it may be made worse. The relief of pain by recumbency is due to removing part of the strain caused by movement or muscle action in trying to maintain the upright position. The increase of pain in recumbency occurs if the body weight in the supine position imposes an increased strain on the back muscles. It is in such cases that immobilization of the back is necessary in addition to bed rest. This type of low back pain is more common among men than among women.

Cases of low back pain in which there is no tightness of low back muscles, but in which alignment is very faulty, are, on the contrary, more common among women than among men. The fault is often associated with weakness of the abdominal muscles. The onset of symptoms is usually gradual rather than acute, and symptoms often remain more or less chronic. Pain is less if the person is active than if he is standing still. It is relieved by recumbency or sitting.

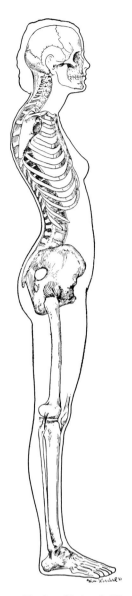

FIG. 125. Faulty Skeletal Alignment

The outline for the above illustration was reproduced from the photograph seen in fig. 10. The faulty positions assumed by the spine, pelvis, head, and chest in such a posture are indicated by this anatomical drawing of the skeletal structure.

There are various types of postural and muscle faults associated with lumbo-sacral strain. Differences are best discussed under three classifications based on faults in pelvic alignment. Symptoms of pain and the constancy of these symptoms vary greatly with the different alignment faults and muscle imbalances which are present.

ANTERIOR PELVIC TILT OR LORDOSIS POSTURE

This type of posture involves an undue compression stress on the posterior part of the vertebral bodies and on the articulating facets. There is undue tension on the anterior vertebral ligament in the lumbar region. (See fig. 125) The muscle imbalances most frequently associated with an anterior tilt may be any one or all of the following:

> Tight low back muscles
> Weak abdominal muscles
> Tight hip flexor muscles
> Weak hamstring muscles

TIGHT LOW BACK MUSCLES. The fault associated with a lordosis posture and tightness of low back muscles is often referred to as a "weak back". The term is applied because of the aching feeling and fatigue that accompanies it, and because of the inability to lift heavy objects without pain. This type of back is mechanically weak and inefficient, but the back muscles are not weak. They are strong, overdeveloped, and short. Use of the term "weak" in connection with such a back often mistakenly carries the connotation that the muscles are weak and that they are in need of strengthening exercises. The term *weak back* would be more aptly applied to the relatively rare type in which the muscles actually are weak and the back is flat or in a position of lumbar kyphosis.

The lordosis posture with tight back muscles tends to give rise to pain in movement or position. Change of position of the body does not give much relief if tightness is severe. The back remains "immobilized" in faulty alignment by this muscle tightness whether the individual is standing, sitting, or lying.

Treatment requires that the tight muscles be stretched to permit a correction of the faulty alignment, but if there has been an acute onset of symptoms associated with severe strain of the back muscles, specific therapy aimed at correction of the underlying fault must wait until acute symptoms have subsided. Healing is promoted by immobilization in a position that relieves tension on the strained muscles and, for that reason, little if any correction of the lordosis can be made until the acute pain has subsided. (See figures 116, 118, and 120 for types of support used in cases of acute low back pain.)

Treatment indications for correction of the low back muscle tightness:

1. Heat and massage to low back

   The patient lies prone on the table with the feet extending over the end of the table and a rolled blanket under the ankles to relieve tension posteriorly on the knee joint. A pillow is placed directly under the abdomen to flex the lumbar spine. (Care should be taken in placing the pillow. If it is too far down under the hips or too far up under the chest, it will hyperextend rather than flex the lumbar spine.) Heat of moderate degree is applied to the low back for fifteen to twenty minutes. Then the low back muscles are massaged, beginning, if necessary, with a rather light stroking but increasing, after several treatments, to a heavier deep kneading to soften and stretch the tight lumbo-sacral muscles and fascia. The patient's tolerance as shown by treatment reaction must be the guide in determining the increase in amount and intensity of the massage. Very little thumb friction is used because it frequently irritates and causes the muscles to tighten rather than to relax.

2. Stretching of the low back muscles

   Carefully graduated exercises and stretching are used. Cases differ and exercises are modified accordingly. Heat and massage always precede stretching. Most of the following exercises are done four or five times during the first treatments and are gradually increased in number to eight or ten times by the end of two weeks.

   Prone with a pillow under the abdomen: Have the patient roll his pelvis over the pillow by pulling down posteriorly with the hamstrings and the gluteals to flatten the lumbar spine and stretch the low back muscles. (See exercise sheet p. 114.)

   Sitting on table with legs extended: The knees are allowed to flex slightly by placing a rolled blanket under them so that in forward bending the tension on the hamstrings is relieved. The patient then reaches down toward the toes pulling up-and-in strongly with the abdominal muscles and down with the buttocks. The movement may rather crudely be described as making the effort to "sit on the end of the spine" as in a slumped position, while, at the same time, reaching forward toward the toes. This movement, if done properly, localizes the stretching to the low back muscles without any stretching to the hamstrings. If the back is quite rigid, additional massage is given while the patient is bending forward.

   A more vigorous stretching of the low back muscles is accomplished in the following manner: the patient sits on a table with legs extended forward and with a rolled blanket under his knees. A wide strap or a folded sheet is placed across the lower abdomen and pulled backward so that the the pelvis is held back and prevented from completely flexing on the thighs. The therapist pushes forward with pressure at the low dorsal region and the patient bends forward pulling in with his abdominal muscles to obtain as much active flexion of the low back as possible.

The following exercises are contra-indicated:

   Hyperextension exercises of the low back from prone position, or double leg-raising, or "sit-ups" in which the back is permitted to hyperextend. (See analysis pp. 50, 51 and 54 for reasons.)

It is an important part of treatment to curtail occupational or recreational activities which require strenuous use of the back during the painful and early corrective stage.

It is not uncommon to find that patients complain of a feeling of unusual fatigue, or even a feeling of nausea for a while after beginning the stretching of the low back. They frequently attribute it to pressure of the pillow under the abdomen, while lying prone, but apparently it comes from low back stretching whether or not this position is used in treatment.

A type of support designed to aid in restoring normal alignment of the spine may be indicated if the tightness is severe and resistant to treatment. Such a support maintains a constant tension on the low back muscles by its pull in the direction of correcting the lordosis. (See fig. 117)

During the stage in which the muscles are tight the individual may be less comfortable on a firm mattress than on a soft one which conforms to his fault. As the tightness is relieved and the mobility restored in the back, he will obtain more comfort from a firm mattress.

WEAK ABDOMINAL MUSCLES. The individual with a lordosis type posture in which abdominal weakness is present (without tightness of the back) usually complains of symptoms across the low back. In early stages it is described as fatigue, and later as an ache, which may or may not become acutely painful. It is usually worse at the end of a day, but is relieved by recumbency to such an extent that after a night's rest the individua may be free of symptoms. He is most comfortable sleeping on a firm mattress because the low back tends to flatten against a flat mattress and this change from a lordosis gives comfort to the back. The position may be eased by sitting if he sits resting against the back of a chair and does not try to sit erect.

If low back muscle tightness is present along with the abdominal muscle weakness, the symptoms and treatment indications are complicated by the factors described above in relation to the tightness.

Treatment indications for correction of abdominal muscle weakness:

1. Treatment to correct tightness of opposing muscles, namely, low back extensors or hip flexors.
2. Application of a support to relieve tension on the weak abdominals. (See figs. 117, 118, and 120) It should be necessary to continue wearing the support only until strength of muscles is good, specifically having a grade of about 80 per cent. (See muscle testing, pp. 79–81.)
3. Exercises. (The choice of exercises depends on the test findings.)

If weakness is present in the "lower" abdominal muscles the following two exercises are indicated:

a. In the back-lying position, place a rolled blanket or small pillow under the knees. With hands up beside the head, tilt the pelvis to flatten the low back on the table by pulling up and in with the lower abdominal muscles. Hold the back flat and breathe in and out easily, relaxing the upper abdominal muscles. There should be good chest expansion during inspiration, but the back should not arch.

b. In the back-lying position, bend the knees and place the feet flat on the table. With the hands up beside the head, tilt the pelvis to flatten the low back on the table. Hold the back flat and slide the heels down along the table. Straighten the legs as much as possible with the back held flat. Keep the back flat and return the knees to the bent position sliding one leg back at a time. (See fig. 126 A, B, C.)

A patient with weak abdominals but with a flexible back will usually do the pelvic tilt movement quite easily. In a patient with very tight low back and hip flexor muscles, the movement of tilting the pelvis to flatten the lumbar spine is prevented by the tight muscles, and the feeling of "rolling the pelvis" cannot be obtained unless the hips are slightly flexed. An assistant aids the patient to rotate the pelvis posteriorly. If treatment to correct accompanying muscle tightness is being given, the patient should soon accomplish the movement of flattening the lum-

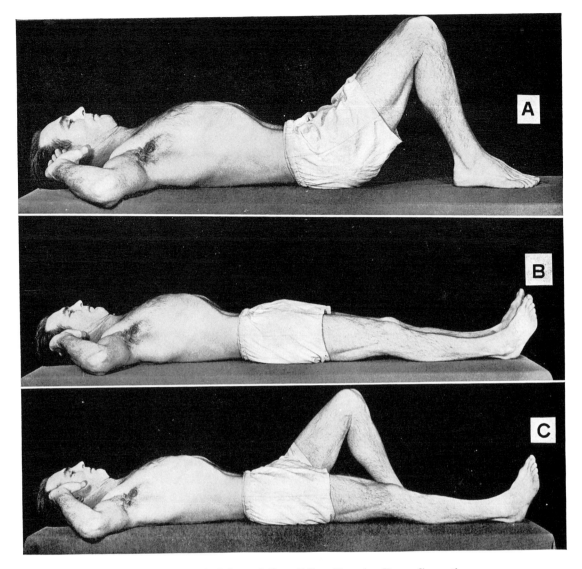

FIG. 126. Pelvic Tilt and Leg-sliding Exercise Done Correctly
(See description of exercise in text p. 128)

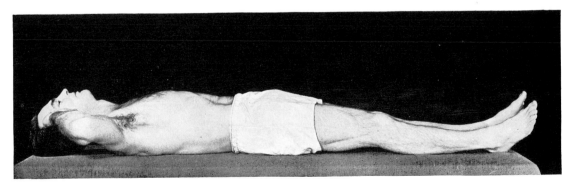

FIG. 127. Incorrect Way of Doing Pelvic Tilt Exercise

bar spine on the table without the necessity of flexing the hips.

If weakness is present in the "upper" abdominal muscles, *and* if there is no kyphosis which would contra-indicate the use of trunk flexion movements, the following exercise is indicated:

In the back-lying position, tilt the pelvis to flatten the low back on the table. With arms extended forward, raise the head and shoulders about eight inches up from the table. Do not attempt to come to a sitting position but raise the upper trunk as high as the back will bend. (See exercise sheet p. 114.) The following exercises are contra-indicated:

Double-leg raising exercise. (See p.50.)

"Sit-ups" with feet hooked under support and done with "chest leading".

Incorrect pelvic tilt exercise. (See fig. 127.)

The rectus abdominis should not act along with the external oblique.

Abdominal muscle weakness is present for varying lengths of time following pregnancy. Being cognizant of this fact a physician often gives his patients a list of exercises at the time of discharge. Some of these exercises presumably should help strengthen the abdominal muscles. Unfortunately these lists often include double-leg raising and "sit-ups", two exercises which should not be given.

TIGHT HIP FLEXOR MUSCLES. Tightness of hip flexors may cause as serious a problem of faulty alignment as weakness of the abdominals or tightness of the back. However, the fault will not give rise to such acute problems of muscle strain as does back tightness because more of the everyday activities put tension on back muscles than on hip flexors. Hip flexor tightness may exist without back tightness and vice versa, but often they are found in combination.

Tightness of hip flexors tends to cause a position of lordosis in standing. Pain may be relieved in sitting because tension on the tight muscles is relieved by the hip flexion and the back may assume a good alignment. At the same time, continuous sitting, such as some occupations require, aggravates this fault by permitting adaptive shortening of these muscles.

There is difficulty in overcoming hip flexor tightness by occasional periods of treatment if one must stay in a sitting position during his occupational activities. The patient should realize that it may be necessary to do stretching every day to try to counteract the factor of continuous sitting.

The individual who has hip flexor tightness can usually find comfort in the lying position by flexing the hips and knees slightly. A firm mattress gives more relief than a soft one which permits the weight of the hips to pull the pelvis into an anterior tilt even though knees are bent.

The individual with lordosis due to hip flexor tightness does not have restriction in forward bending as does the one with back tightness.

Treatment indications for correction of hip flexor tightness:

1. Heat and massage to antero-lateral thigh.
2. Stretching of tight hip flexors. (See exercise sheet p. 115.)

The following exercises are contra-indicated:

Hip flexion exercises such as single or double leg-raising.

"Sit-ups" with feet hooked under support.

WEAK HAMSTRING MUSCLES. In the anterior pelvic tilt type of faulty posture, hamstring weakness is a less constant finding than the three imbalances previously described. It is seldom found as a primary factor, but when it is found in conjunction with abdominal weakness, the pelvic tilt and lordosis tend to be more exaggerated than if such weakness were not present. Ordinary sitting with knees bent relieves tension on the hamstrings and this may account for the fact that these muscles are not as consistently weak as the abdominals in lordosis postures.

Standing with knees hyperextended and pelvis tilted anteriorly puts tension on hamstrings, causing gradually increasing stretch-weakness of these muscles.

In the standing position, hamstring muscles feel *taut* whether they are stretched or contracted. Usually this tautness is interpreted as contracted hamstrings on postural inspection, with the result that treatment to stretch hamstrings is ordered as a corrective measure. When this tautness is associated with stretched hamstrings, stretching is contra-indicated. Accurate examination for hamstring length (as described in Chap. IV) is necessary for accurate diagnosis, and for prescription of therapeutic measures.

It is not practical to apply a support to correct knee-hyperextension in the ordinary postural cases. The subject must be trained to correct this fault voluntarily by changing the habitual position of his knees in standing.

Correction of the anterior pelvic tilt by whatever measures are indicated by the examination findings, will also relieve tension on the hamstrings. After treatment has been instituted for relief of tension, exercise to strengthen these muscles is indicated. Standing or lying pelvic tilt exercise with emphasis on pulling the pelvis down posteriorly is used for strengthening the hamstrings. Resisted knee flexion exercises in sitting may be used, but the exercise of knee flexion from a prone position involves too much back fixation to make it therapeutic in most cases of anterior pelvic tilt.

POSTERIOR PELVIC TILT

Two types of postural problems appear in connection with posterior pelvic tilt. One is that in which the back is flat and the low back muscles are tight and over-developed, giving rise to a rigid, flat-back posture. The lumbo-sacral strain associated with such a fault is usually one of acute strain of the low back muscles occurring during a forward bending movement. The movement which causes the onset may appear trivial or may be one of over-exertion. Palliative and corrective treatment for the muscle strain and tightness are essentially the same as for the low back tightness described above under anterior pelvic tilt. In regard to alignment, however, an effort should be made to obtain an increase rather than a decrease in the lumbar curve, that is, a more nearly normal alignment of the lumbar spine. Further details in regard to this type of fault are discussed below under "Sacro-iliac strain".

The second type of problem in relation to posterior pelvic tilt is that of a *weak back* in which the back and hip flexor muscles are weak and the lumbar spine is either flat or in slight

kyphosis. This type of back is relatively uncommon, but when it exists it offers a serious problem in faulty mechanics.

In standing, sitting, and forward bending there is the element of undue compression on the anterior surfaces of the bodies of the lumbar vertebrae, and constant tension on the muscles and posterior spinous ligaments of the low back. The constant muscle tension may give rise to symptoms of strain and fatigue that may become quite acute. The greatest strain may be felt in the dorso-lumbar region in sitting because the compensatory forward inclination of the upper trunk puts the greatest stress at this junction.

Weakness of hip flexors, particularly the psoas major, is one of the most constant findings in cases of posterior pelvic tilt with lumbar kyphosis. Primary weakness of these muscles may give rise to the fault, or stretch-weakness of these muscles may gradually occur due to the faulty alignment.

Treatment requires a support which holds the spine in good mechanical position, i.e., in a normal anterior curve of the lumbar spine. Correction should not be forced, but attempts should be made to accomplish gradually an improvement in alignment. Best results will be obtained by constant wearing of the support for sitting or standing positions. If symptoms have reached the acute stage, a support should be worn while recumbent, also, until acute symptoms subside.

After strain and fatigue have been relieved by the support, exercises for the low back and hip flexor muscles are indicated. Hyperextension exercises are indicated for the back. For the hip flexors, alternate leg-raising from the supine position is usually a suitable exercise. Though the back should not be allowed to arch abnormally, it should be allowed to arch slightly during the alternate leg-raising because, in giving this exercise, the objective is to strengthen the psoas so that it will exert a pull forward on the lumbar spine. Double leg-raising is liable to be too strenuous a movement, so it is not recommended.

The posture of one with hip flexor weakness is that of hip hyperextension, the pelvis and upper end of the femur being deviated forward in the same manner that the lower end of the femur and upper end of the tibia and fibula deviate backward in knee-hyperextension. Correction of the faulty postural alignment in standing is done by training in much the same manner, and for the same reason as in correcting knee-hyperextension.

LATERAL PELVIC TILT

The low back pain associated with lateral pelvic tilt appears as a unilateral lumbo-sacral strain.

As many (if not more) of the problems of postural low back pain are associated with lateral pelvic tilt as with anterior pelvic tilt. The mechanical problem is chiefly that of undue compression at the articulating facets of the spine on the high side of the pelvis. The sore spot which corresponds with the area of greatest compression is over the articulating facet of the fifth lumbar on the high side.

Since most right-handed people exhibit the pattern of faulty mechanics in which the hip is higher on the right than on the left, unilateral lumbo-sacral strains occur more often on the right than on the left, with the painful area to the right of the 5th lumbar vertebra.

Muscle imbalances are usually present in the lateral or postero-lateral trunk, and the lateral or antero-lateral thigh muscles in the cases of lateral pelvic tilt. The postero-lateral trunk muscles and lumbo-dorsal fascia are tighter on the high side of the pelvis while the leg abductors and tensor fascia lata are tighter on the low side of the pelvis. The abductors, particularly the posterior part of the gluteus medius, show weakness on the high side while the leg on this side assumes a position of postural adduction in relation to the pelvis. (See fig. 76.) An imbalance may also be noted in the hip adductors. The pattern most frequently seen in right-handed individuals is that of tight left tensor, weak right gluteus medius, stronger hip adductors and lateral trunk muscles on the right than on the left.

Left-handed individuals tend to show the reverse of this pattern. Facilities and equipment are most often made for right-handed use if there is an element of asymmetry involved in activity. Left-handed people are, therefore, often required to use tools or equipment in a right-handed manner, with the result that acquired patterns of muscle imbalances tend to be less fixed than in the right-handed individuals.

As a result of the faulty lateral alignment and the muscle imbalances, pain may appear in the low back or in the leg. Usually careful examination will show some evidence of symptoms in both of these areas regardless of the area of chief complaint.

When pain is most evident in the low back the lumbo-sacral irritation is basically one of undue compression. Treatment is primarily concerned with re-alignment to relieve such compression. Essentially, treatment consists of the application of a straight raise on the heel of the shoe on the low side of the pelvis, i.e., the side opposite the low back compression. Because unilateral lumbo-sacral strain is more often on the right, the straight raise is usually required on the left. Seldom is it necessary or advisable to use a lift thicker than $\frac{1}{8}''$ or $\frac{3}{16}''$. A firm rubber and leather heel pad that can be inserted into a shoe often suffices.

Obviously, it is not to be assumed that a lift may be applied indiscriminately on the left side. The difference in level of the posterior spines as seen with the patient standing should provide the basis for determining the need for, and the amount of, shoe lift. Findings may be confirmed by measurements of x-rays taken with the patient standing if that is desired. The muscle test findings relating to gluteus medius strength (see p. 89) should be used to confirm the diagnosis in regard to the "apparent leg length difference". Apparent leg length measurements taken in the supine position for use as a basis in determining the side of application of the lift are, unfortunately, more often misleading than not. (See analysis of fallacy in this regard, p. 97.)

If there is tightness in the tensor fascia lata on one side, the faulty alignment will not automatically be corrected by the application of a shoe lift. It is necessary to treat this tightness even though no specific symptoms are present in that area. Such treatment should either precede or accompany the use of the shoe lift. (See p. 137 regarding specific treatment of the tight fascia.)

The weakness of the gluteus medius, which is usually present on the high side of the pelvis, must be corrected so the medius can better help maintain lateral alignment. The shoe correction which is used to level the pelvis at once removes the element of tension on the weaker medius and the exercise involved in the ordinary functional activity of walking suffices for strengthening this muscle. It has not been found necessary to give added exercise for leg abduction to individuals who are normally active.

A minimum of six weeks is advised for wearing the lift. Whether it is needed longer depends, to a great extent, on how long the immediate postural problem has existed, whether any actual leg length difference exists, and whether occupational activities or postural habits can be changed to permit maintenance of good alignment.

Though it may be slight, some degree of rotation of the pelvis on the femora accompanies a lateral pelvic tilt. The rotation appears to follow the pattern set by the lateral tilt of the pelvis rather than being established in direct relationship to the muscle imbalance. The pelvis tends to rotate forward on the side of a high hip. In other words, there usually is counter-clockwise rotation of the pelvis when the right hip is high and the right leg is in postural adduction on the pelvis. The rotation tends to disappear when the pelvis is leveled laterally.

Sacro-Iliac Strain

From the standpoint of mechanics, a sacro-iliac strain is chiefly one of *undue tension* on the ligaments supporting this joint. No muscles specifically reinforce the sacro-iliac joint, but associated muscle problems do exist.

In the more typical cases of sacro-iliac strain the posture is one of a flat back in which the low back and hamstring muscles are tight. The tight low back muscles and lumbo-dorsal fascia pulling upward on the sacrum, and the tight hamstring muscles and posterior thigh (gluteal) fascia pulling downward on the pelvis, exert stresses in opposite directions producing tension on the sacro-iliac joint. The opposing stresses may exert some tension when the body is upright, but exert their greatest tension during forward bending movements.

Tightness of the back holds the sacrum and lumbar spine as a fixed immobile unit. Tightness of the posterior thigh muscles and fascia maintain a fixed relationship of the pelvis and leg as soon as movement in flexion has progressed to the limit of range permitted by the short muscles.

When movement in flexion of the back and hip joints is at the maximum afforded by the muscle length, the muscles of the back or legs or the ligaments of the sacro-iliac joint are subject to strain. Where the strain will occur depends on the resistance of these structures. Thus it is that either a lumbo-sacral or a sacro-iliac strain may occur in this type posture, or the two may occur simultaneously.

It is quite generally assumed that the ligaments of the sacro-iliac joint are so strong and movement so limited that a strain is not likely to occur except by severe injury. Anatomists agree, however, that this joint does permit some motion. It is called a diarthrosis rather than a synchrondrosis. Because the normal range of motion of the joint is small, it takes very little more to be excessive. A tension sufficient to cause ligamentous strain may not appear as a visible separation on x-ray.

Among women the most frequent cause of a sacro-iliac strain is child-birth. There is normally some relaxation of the ligaments at this time, and the stress of delivery occasionally causes severe strain on this joint.

In men sacro-iliac strain occurs most frequently among laborers engaged in heavy lifting. The occupation of the laborer often requires a partially bent position of the knees and a partially bent position of the spine for the motion and strength of lifting. He uses his back muscles in strenuous movements, but may seldom move into a position of hyperextension of the back because it is so inefficient mechanically for lifting heavy weights. The hamstrings remain in a relatively shortened position and in use most of the time during such activity. The back muscles while not favored by being in a shortened position are not under undue tension or stretch, and, being in constant use, become short from over-development.

Sacro-iliac strain may occur in patients with a lordosis posture who have tightness of the back muscles, but such cases are less common than among the flat-back postures.

Sacro-iliac strain may be bilateral or unilateral. It may exist in conjunction with a unilateral lumbo-sacral strain on the opposite side. As such the combination occurs most frequently as a right lumbo-sacral, and a left sacro-iliac strain.

Correction of faulty mechanics associated with sacro-iliac strain depends on the specific faults in alignment and muscle imbalance that are present. Since these vary, examination for tightness, weakness, or alignment faults should be made before prescribing treatment.

Hamstring tightness is one of the more constant findings in this type of postural fault, and should be treated by the application of heat, massage, and stretching movements.

A position of straight-leg-raising from a back-lying position puts tension on the hamstrings. It is difficult, however, when treating hamstrings to apply the principle that the tight muscles should be under slight tension during the application of heat. For convenience, the patient lies prone on the table during the application of heat. During the massage, he is placed in a back-lying position, and, instead of having the leg held up in a position of straight-leg-raise by an assistant, the foot rests against a wall for support. This puts the leg in a position of hamstring stretch. The patient's other knee must be bent to permit him to get as close as possible to the wall. A stroking and kneading massage to the hamstrings is done with the patient in this position. As the muscles relax, the patient moves closer to the wall and the leg is raised higher to give added stretch to the hamstrings. It would

be desirable that the opposite leg be extended, but this is difficult unless some other set-up is used. When passive stretching is done at home a patient may substitute a chair-back for the wall. He may lie on the floor with one leg out straight beside the chair while the other is in a position of straight-leg-raise resting the foot against the chair-back.

If the low back muscles are short as in the rigid flat-back posture, heat, massage, and stretching of the low back muscles are indicated and should be applied in the same manner as for a tight lordotic back. (See p. 127.) Since range of motion in hyperextension is also limited in the rigid flat-back posture, there is a temptation to prescribe hyperextension exercises. Movement in the direction of hyperextension is indicated, but active exercise of the contracted low back muscles is not. Increased range in extension of the spine should be obtained by passive movements, such as lying in a supine position with a small pillow under the back for short periods of time.

Supportive treatment consists chiefly of a sacro-iliac belt. If there has been a lumbo-sacral strain in conjunction with the sacro-iliac strain, a corset or back brace is indicated also. The sacro-iliac belt is then incorporated with the support. (See figs. 118 and 119.)

In case of sacro-iliac strain, pain is less in standing than in sitting. Forward bending causes more pain. There tends also to be pain referred to the lower anterior abdominal region, and there may be associated sciatic symptoms.

Facet-Slipping

The joints or facets which connect one vertebra with another may show abnormal deviations of alignment, referred to as a facet-slipping. Conceivably, a slipping may occur at the limit of range in flexion or in hyperextension.

As a fault in hyperextension it may result from either a sudden movement in that direction, or from a severe and persistent lumbar lordosis. The latter has been seen in x-ray.[*]

* Paul C. Williams, M.D.: Lesions of the Lumbosacral Spine. Part II. Chronic Traumatic (Postural) Destruction of the Lumbosacral Intervertebral Disc, The Journal of Bone and Joint Surgery, July, 1937, p. 690.

The vertebral interspaces are diminished and the lordosis is so marked that the compression force has caused joint structures to give way and permit the "over-riding" of one facet on another.

The suddenness of onset, acuteness of pain, and absence of previous neuromuscular symptoms lead to the supposition that some cases of acute low back pain may be due to facet-slipping. The patient's description of "hearing a click like something slipping out of place" suggests that an alignment fault had occurred. Usually these incidents are of momentary duration, and as such are not confirmed by x-ray. The diagnosis necessarily is based on subjective rather than objective findings.

The movement of the body, and the direction of stress denote the direction of the alignment fault. Most often it occurs during flexion and the patient says he "couldn't straighten up." The complaint is not unlike that following severe strain of the muscles, however.

As a fault in flexion the slipping would be more apt to occur in the very flexible back, while the muscle strain more often occurs in the tight back.

In strong hyperextension movements the so-called "catch in the back" may be purely muscle spasm or may involve excessive motion in the form of facet-slipping.

The faults of alignment and mobility which result in excessive joint motion are the basic factors to be considered in correcting or preventing faults of this type.

Coccyalgia

Coccyalgia or coccygodynia refers to pain in the coccyx or neighboring area. Numerous factors including trauma are responsible for coccyalgia. Though faulty position of the body may have no relation to the onset of symptoms, it may result secondarily and become an important factor.

One who has persistent coccyalgia tends to sit in a very erect position with hyperextension (lordosis) of the spine in an effort to avoid undue pressure on the painful coccyx. Years of sitting in such a position, in many instances, result in weakening of the gluteus maximum muscles as revealed by muscle testing.

Conservative treatment consists of applying a back-lace corset that draws the buttocks close together as the straps or laces are tightened. The corset should be drawn tight while the patient is in the standing position. The gluteal muscles thus form a padding for the coccyx in the sitting position. Pain is often alleviated by this simple procedure.

Leg Pain

The conditions discussed under this heading include pain associated with Tensor Fascia Lata Tightness and Sciatica.

Pain associated with Tensor Fascia Lata Tightness

A condition often mistakenly referred to as sciatica is that of pain associated with a contracted tensor fascia lata. Pain may be limited to the area covered by the fascia along the lateral surface of the thigh or may extend upward over the buttocks involving the gluteal fascia as well. Palpation over the full length of the fascia lata from its origin on the iliac crest to the insertion of the ilio-tibial band elicits pain or tenderness. It is especially tender along the upper margin of the trochanter, and at the point of insertion near the head of the fibula.

Painful symptoms may be limited to the area of the thigh or there may exist, along with this syndrome, an irritation of the peroneal nerve. A review of the anatomy of the lateral aspect of the knee shows the relationship of the peroneal nerve to the muscles and fascia in this area. (See fig. 128.)

The peroneal branch of the sciatic nerve passes obliquely forward over the neck of the fibula, crossing directly under the fibers of origin of the peroneus longus muscle. It is well known that any prolonged pressure over this area, even though slight, must be avoided because of the danger of peroneal nerve paralysis. Even in the application of adhesive traction to the lower leg one must be extremely cautious to avoid either *pressure* over the nerve or *excessive* traction on the soft tissue at that point.

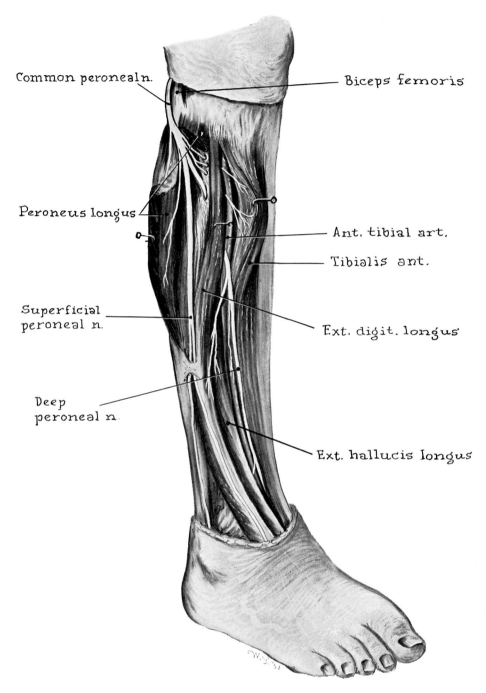

FIG. 128. Relationship of Peroneal Nerve to Neck of Fibula and Peroneus Longus Muscle

The mechanism by which the peroneal nerve is irritated in cases of tightness of the fascia lata may be explained on the basis of either the effect of pressure by the rigid bands of fascia or by the effects of traction on this part. When the tight fascia is drawn taut as in movements of walking, or on movements of testing for tightness, the fascia is often observed to be extremely rigid. The peroneal nerve, crossing under this taut band and lying in close contact with the neck of the fibula, is subjected to constant irritation.

The effect of the element of traction is often seen in acute cases. With the patient lying on his side with the affected leg uppermost, the mere dropping of the foot into inversion by the pull of gravity (downward toward the table), puts tension on the muscles and fascial bands. Symptoms of nerve irritation are often elicited in the area supplied by the peroneal nerve by this simple movement of the foot.

The failure to recognize the peripheral cause of this peroneal nerve irritation has often resulted in rather obscure explanations of this syndrome.

Often deduction that the pain was due to nerve root lesion has been based on the fact that the dermatome area of cutaneous distribution corresponds so closely to the area of pain when the peroneal nerve is involved.

Patterns of faulty mechanics bear a close relationship to handedness. Most people stand with the right hip higher than the left. The tensor fascia is thereby more often contracted on the left than on the right, and most cases of unilateral tensor pain appear in the left leg. Chronic sciatic symptoms associated with faulty posture appear more often on the right. (See discussion under sciatica below.) Symptoms of tensor pain are more common than those of chronic sciatica.

Tensor pain may be bilateral or unilateral, but is more often unilateral if severe. The effect of being bilateral is self-limiting in the extent of the imbalance that can arise. Activities such as skating, skiing, or horse-back riding may predispose, however, toward tightness of the tensor on both right and left.

TREATMENT INDICATIONS

FOR ACUTE SYMPTOMS. Heat is applied to the lateral aspect of the thigh while the patient is in a position that "gives in" to the tightness. This is done by abducting the leg in back-lying or side-lying. To support the leg in abduction in side-lying, a firm pillow is placed between the thighs and another between the lower legs, making sure that the foot is supported also in this side-lying position. A pillow at the back or abdomen helps balance the patient comfortably in this side-lying position. Heat may be applied two or three times a day for about 20 to 30 minute periods while the patient remains in bed.

As soon as the patient can tolerate it, which may be during the first treatment or may be two or three days later, massage may be started. Massage should be *firm* but not deep. Often a very superficial stroking is more irritating than a firm gentle pressure in cases of tensor pain. The patients frequently describe the reaction to the massage as "a hurt that feels good" They are aware of a feeling of tightness and describe it as "wishing they could make the muscle let go" or that "it would feel good if somebody stretched it".

The almost immediate relief of symptoms indicates that the condition is basically one of tight muscles and fascia. These treatment-reactions differ from those in sciatica. The same procedures applied to the painful area along the hamstring muscles in cases of sciatic irritation would give rise to increased pain. The patient should avoid exposure to cold or drafts because even the slightest exposure often causes aggravation until acute symptoms subside.

FOR SUB-ACUTE STAGES. As acute pain subsides, succeeding treatments should be directed toward stretching the tight fascia. During treatment, abduction of the thigh is gradually diminished until it is in a position of slight tension on the abductors while the heat and massage are applied. The position and movement for stretching are illustrated on p. 115 on the exercise sheet.

Self stretching in the standing position (as first described by Dr. Frank Ober*) may be done if the pelvis is kept from any anterior tilt as this movement is performed.

The shoe correction, which is indicated for the correction of the lateral pelvic tilt associated with tensor fascia lata tightness, acts also as an aid in the gradual stretching of the tight fascia. For this reason, such shoe alterations may not be tolerated until acute symptoms have subsided, and until some active treatment, in the form of heat and massage, has been instituted to relax and stretch the tight fascia.

Though the condition of pain associated with a contracted tensor fascia lata is the more common, there are instances of *strain* on the high side of the pelvis. When a leg is in a position of marked postural adduction, there is a continuous tension on the abductors of the thigh on that side. The symptoms may become quite acute. If present they are treated by relief of strain—that is, leveling the pelvis and correction of any opposing muscle tightness which may be causing the persistent tension. Since the chief opponent is the opposite tensor, this problem resolves itself into treatment of the contracted muscles and fascia on the low side, even though symptoms of strain are present on the other side.

Sciatica

Sciatica refers to a neuritic type of pain along the course of the sciatic nerve. Pain extends down the posterior thigh and lower leg to the sole of the foot, and along the lateral aspect of the lower leg to the dorsum of the foot.

Sciatica may occur in connection with various infections or inflammatory disease processes, or may be due to some mechanical factor of compression, tension, or irritation.

The symptoms may originate from a lesion of one or more of the nerve roots which later join through a plexus to form the sciatic nerve. A protruded intervertebral disc is an example of mechanical irritation that is present at the

* Ober, F. R.: Back Strain and Sciatica, J. A. M. A. 104: 1580 (May 4) 1935.

level where the nerve roots emerge from the spinal canal. Distribution of pain tends to extend from the root origin to the terminal nerve endings with the result that it is quite widespread. An L5 lesion, for example, may give rise, not only to symptoms down the course of the sciatic nerve, but also to pain in the region of the posterior and lateral thigh supplied by the inferior and superior gluteal nerves.

Symptoms of sciatica may arise from irritation anywhere along the course of the sacral plexus, the sciatic nerve trunk, or its peripheral nerve branches. Sciatica may arise as reflex pain from irritation of peripheral nerve endings. Unless so severe as to set up a reflex mechanism, a lesion along the course of the nerve or its branches may often be distinguished from a root lesion by the localization of pain to the distribution below the level of the lesion.

Other than at the root, there are two commonly recognized sites of lesions giving rise to sciatic pain: 1) the sacro-iliac region where the spinal nerves emerge through the sacral foramen; 2) at the level of the piriformis muscle where the sciatic nerve trunk emerges through the sciatic notch.

This discussion about sciatica will be concerned with faulty body mechanics in relation to disc protrusion, and the sciatic symptoms associated with the piriformis syndrome. There will be no discussion of sciatica in relation to sacro-iliac strain other than to suggest that the faulty mechanics causing this strain (as described above) may put tension on the sacral plexus because of the close association of the involved structures in this area.

PROTRUDED INTERVERTEBRAL DISC

Sciatica resulting from a ruptured disc has been described in elaborate detail in the literature. In such a lesion, surgery for removal of the disc is usually indicated. It would not be logical to assume that conservative treatment could effect any permanent relief of symptoms caused by a fixed protrusion of a disc. There are cases of sciatica, however, in which clinical findings suggest a disc lesion, but the fluctuation or inconstancy of symptoms suggest that the protrusion is not constant. Conservative treatment of many such cases has brought about effective relief of symptoms without surgery, previous to and since the advent of surgical treatment for this lesion.

There are instances in which, for some reason, the patient declines operation or the doctor does not elect to do surgery. Conservative treatment is the necessary alternative.

The rationale of conservative treatment is based on the supposition that any compressive force whether due to muscle spasm or tightness of the back muscles, or the stress of the superimposed weight of the trunk on the lumbar spine, may be a factor in causing disc protrusion.

To this end, two measures are necessary in effective conservative treatment: first, immobilization of the back for relief of any acute muscle spasm; and second, use of a support for the low back which acts to transmit the weight of the thorax to the pelvis and relieve stress on the lumbar spine. In much the same manner, a cervical collar is used to relieve pressure on the cervical spine.

To treat by immobilization, and for relief of compression, a fitted front-lace corset-type support is used. Such a support should be reinforced with strong lateral and posterior stays. (See figs. 118 and 120).

Following relief of acute symptoms, therapeutic measures are instituted to correct any underlying muscle imbalance or faults in alignment.

Acute sciatic symptoms associated with protrusion of a ruptured disc are often described as having occurred as a result of a sudden twist and extension of the spine from a forward bent position such as twisting the trunk while lifting a weight. That such a type of stress should be related to this specific type of lesion is not surprising in view of the fact that (according to Gray) "rotation of the lumbar spine takes place at the intervertebral disc".

The factors of rotation and extension of the lumbar spine are also related to the faulty mechanics observed in cases of chronic sciatica.

Low back muscles are tight, the back may or may not be in a position of lordosis, and there is rotation and unilateral pelvic tilt. Chronic sciatic symptoms occur more frequently on the right than on the left because the usual pattern of faulty body mechanics presents a right high hip and counter-clockwise rotation of the pelvis.

That tensor fascia lata pain occurs more frequently on the left, and the chronic sciatica associated with faulty body mechanics more frequently on the right, may be regarded as of value in the differential diagnosis.

Sciatica which has been acute or sub-acute often causes the body to be drawn into such faulty alignment that symptoms of muscle strain and faulty alignment are added to the original disability. These secondary symptoms may, on occasion, persist after the original causative factors have subsided.

PIRIFORMIS MUSCLE AND ITS RELATION TO SCIATIC PAIN

Dr. Freiberg*, in discussing the piriformis muscle and its relation to sciatic pain, has furnished an interesting explanation regarding a possible cause of sciatic symptoms. Though there may be numerous cases in which sciatic pain is associated with a *contracted* piriformis, as he describes, it is the opinion of the authors that irritation of the sciatic nerve by the piriformis muscle is more often associated with a stretched piriformis.

The piriformis arises with a broad origin from the anterior aspect of the sacrum and inserts into the superior border of the greater trochanter. This muscle has three functions in standing. It acts as an external rotator of the femur, aids slightly in tilting the pelvis down laterally, and aids in tilting the pelvis posteriorly by pulling the sacrum down toward the leg which is the fixed point in standing.

When a faulty mechanical position is present in which a leg is in postural adduction and

* Freiberg, Albert H. and Vinke, Theodore H.: Sciatica and Sacro-Iliac Joint, Journal of Bone and Joint Surgery, Volume XVI: pp. 126-136.

internal rotation in relation to an anteriorly tilted pelvis, there is marked stretching of the piriformis muscle along with other muscles that function in a similar manner. The mechanics of the position are such that the piriformis muscle and the sciatic nerve are thrust into close contact. This is somewhat in contrast to a contracted piriformis muscle in which, as suggested by Schudel, "the contracted muscle may well be in position to bridge and protect the sciatic nerve". See fig. 129 which shows the relationship of the sciatic nerve to the piriformis muscle.

The following points should be considered in diagnosing a probable piriformis irritation (associated with a stretched piriformis).

1. Do the sciatic symptoms diminish or disappear in non-weight bearing?
2. Do internal rotation and adduction of the thigh in the flexed position, with patient supine, increase the sciatic symptoms?
3. Do the symptoms diminish in standing if a straight-raise is placed under the opposite foot?
4. Does the patient seek relief of symptoms by placing the leg in external rotation and abduction, both in the lying and standing positions?

The test movement to place the piriformis on maximum stretch (※2 above) is done in the following manner: The patient is placed supine on a table. The knee and hip of the affected leg are flexed to right angles. Flexion of the knee rules out any confusion with pain due to irritation of the hamstring muscles. The examiner then internally rotates and adducts the thigh passively.

In regard to number 3 above, it has been a frequent clinical observation that, during the course of examination, a lift applied under the foot of the affected side would increase symptoms, while a lift placed under the foot of the unaffected side would give some immediate relief in the affected leg.

Shoe corrections, for cases suggesting irritation due to a stretched rather than a contracted piriformis, consist of a straight raise (usually $\frac{1}{8}$ to $\frac{1}{4}$ inch) on the heel on the *unaffected* side to relieve tension on the abductors of the affected

side; and an inner wedge on the heel on the *affected* side to correct the internal rotation of the leg. Heat, massage, and stretching of low back muscles if they are contracted, abdominal muscle exercise if abdominal weakness is present, and instructions for correcting the faulty position of the pelvis in standing are used as indicated.

Knee Pain

The habitual position of the knee in standing suggests which areas are subjected to undue pressure and which are subjected to undue tension. Symptoms of ligamentous strain are associated with the areas of undue tension, while symptoms of bony compression are more often related to the areas of pressure. The variations in symptoms are best described by discussing each type of fault individually. The combination of faults occurs frequently and in rather fixed patterns. For example, the combination of knee hyperextension, internal rotation, and postural bow-legs is rather common. Internal rotation and slight knock-knee are frequently seen in combination. External rotation is often seen with severe knock-knee.

Internal Rotation

"Internal rotation of the knees" is a phrase used to describe the position of the legs, in standing, in which the patellae face slightly inward rather than straight ahead. It may be due to rotation of the entire leg from the hip to the foot, or may be due to some actual rotation of the shaft of the lower leg in relation to the femur. The latter, often described as external tibial torsion, may appear as internal rotation of the knees when the feet are straight ahead, or as an outflare position of the feet if the knees face forward.

Internal rotation of the knees is often seen as the result of postural hyperextension, or in combination with it. The faulty knee position of internal rotation of the femur with external rotation of the lower leg, along with knee hyperextension has a basis in the stretching of the popliteus muscle. This short firm muscle which acts somewhat as a broad posterior knee joint

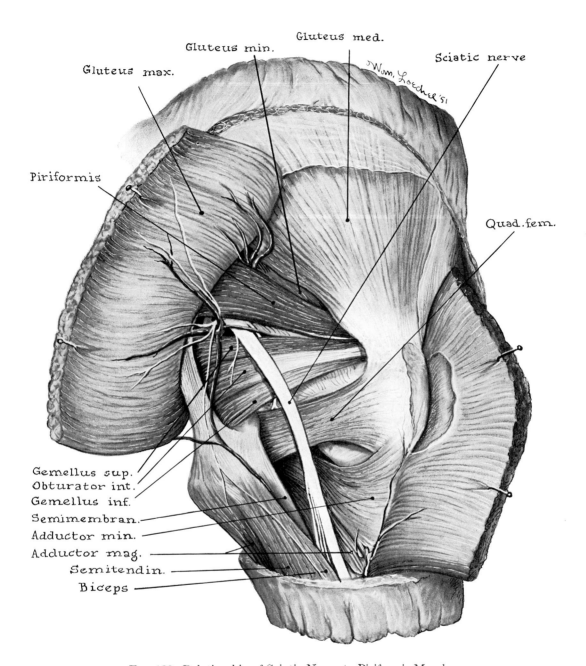

FIG. 129. Relationship of Sciatic Nerve to Piriformis Muscle

ligament, has the function of rotating the lower leg inward on the femur. If it is stretched by knee-hyperextension, it permits the lower leg to rotate outward on the femur. However, this rotation movement can occur only if the knee is flexed or hyperextended because anatomically the knee does not rotate if it is in extension. The remedial treatment for this type of fault is training the person to avoid positions of hyperextension in standing, rather than using any specific exercise or means of support.

Internal rotation of the leg from hip level may result from either or both of the following: weakness of the hip external rotators, or pronation of the foot. Whichever of these predisposes to the fault, the end result is usually that both conditions exist if either is not corrected.

Treatment consists of placing an inner (border) wedge on the heel of the shoe to correct pronation thus helping to rotate the leg back into normal alignment. Shoe correction loses much of its effectiveness if knee alignment is faulty in hyperextension, and if such a fault is present it should have postural correction. Exercises to strengthen the hip rotators and extensors, and correct any faulty pelvic deviation should also be part of the postural correction.

Knock-knee

Tension on the internal lateral ligaments, and compression of the lateral surfaces of the knee joint are present in knock-knee. Pain associated with the postural tension on the ligament is annoying but can be tolerated for a long time before becoming incapacitating. The pain associated with the compression, on the other hand, is slow to develop, but is often intolerable when it manifests itself. Evidence of arthritic changes may appear in x-ray.

In treatment of *mild* knock-knee, an inner border wedge on a shoe tends to re-align the extremity thus relieving strain medially, and compression laterally. There is danger in using too high an inner wedge because the over-correction of the foot may be over-compensated by an increase in the knock-knees. The authors suggest that a $\frac{1}{8}''$ to $\frac{3}{16}''$ inner heel wedge is usually adequate. A *moderate* degree of knock-

knee may be benefited by an elastic knee support in addition to shoe corrections. The support should have lateral steel uprights with a joint at the knee. *Severe* knock-knee requires bracing (as shown in fig. 130) or surgery.

Tightness and soreness of the tensor fascia lata is frequently seen in conjunction with knock-knees, even in young children. Heat, massage and stretching of the fascia is often needed in order that the shoe correction may effectively bring about a realignment.

Knee Hyperextension

The position of postural hyperextension of the knees results in undue compression of the knee joint anteriorly, and undue tension on the ligaments and muscles posteriorly.

Pain in the popliteal space is not uncommon in adults who stand with the knee in hyperextension.

Training in correct postural alignment is the chief form of treatment except in severe cases when a leg brace may be required to prevent hyperextension.

Knee Flexion

The position of knee flexion in standing is less common than the other knee faults discussed above. It may occur in older people but is seldom seen in youngsters, except the unilateral knee flexion which may be compensatory for knock-knee. For the role of hip flexor tightness in postural knee flexion see fig. 44.

Pain is most often associated with muscle strain of the quadriceps, or with the effect of traction by the quadriceps (through its patellar tendon insertion) on the tibia. Painful reactions to this type of fault are seldom seen except in older people and correction is very difficult because of the age of the individual and the established habits of standing.

Bow-legs

In children a position of bow-legs may be either actual or apparent. An actual bowing is of the shaft (femur or tibia or both) and is usually considered to be due to rickets. An apparent bowing occurs as a result of a combination of joint positions permitting the faulty alignment though no actual structural defect is present in the long bones.

The postural bowing is not present if the knees are in a good antero-posterior alignment. Since there is no bony defect, this bowing occurs only if the knee goes into hyperextension or flexion. Thus on testing it will disappear in non-weight bearing or on standing if the knees are held in neutral extension. (See fig. 41.)

Correction depends almost entirely on postural exercises to eliminate the hyperextension. There are numerous instances in which the postural bowing and hyperextension are compensatory for a knock-knee, as discussed on p. 169. Paradoxically the correction of this type of postural bowing must be based on a correction of the underlying knock-knee deformity. (See fig. 147.)

Correction of structural bowing depends chiefly on effective bracing. The brace is made by attaching an inner steel upright to a pelvic band and to a shoe. A wide leather or canvas band, attached to the bar, is so placed that the straps can be drawn tight enough to put traction on the leg, pulling inward toward the straight upright.

An outer wedge on the heel or sole is usually not indicated because of the tendency of the foot to pronate as the legs bow outward.

External Rotation

This fault does not in itself appear to give rise to painful knee conditions. It usually is an expression of outward rotation from hip level, and is accompanied by an out-toeing position of the feet. (See p. 148 and fig. 148.)

Foot Pain

The foot has *two longitudinal arches* which extend lengthwise from the heel to the ball of the foot. The *inner* or *medial* longitudinal arch is made up of the os calcis, astragalus, scaphoid, three cuneiform, and inner three metatarsal bones. The *outer* or *lateral* longitudinal arch is made up of the os calcis, cuboid, and outer two metatarsal bones. The outer arch is lower than the inner and tends to be obliterated in weight bearing. Any reference to "the longitudinal

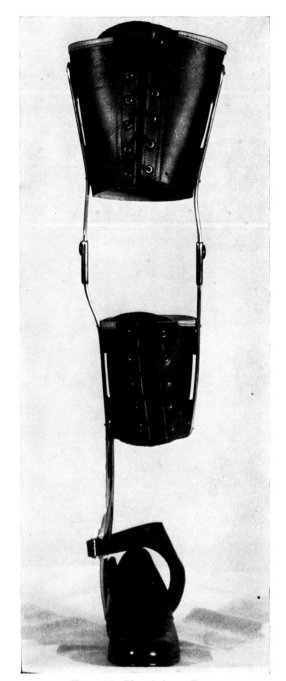

FIG. 130. Knock-knee Brace

In children this type brace may be used to aid in correction of knock-knees; in adults, it is used in cases of pain associated with knock-knees or other faulty knee conditions.

arch" will mean the inner arch; if intended to designate the outer it will be so modified.

There are two *transverse metatarsal arches*, one across the mid section and one across he ball of the foot. The *posterior metatarsal* arch is at the proximal end (or base) of the metatarsal bones. It is a structural arch with wedge shaped bones at the apex of the arch. The *anterior metatarsal* arch is at the distal end (or heads) of the metatarsals. It is an arch which disappears in weight bearing.

Painful foot conditions may be divided, roughly, into three groups, those dealing with longitudinal arch strain, those dealing with metatarsal arch strain, and those dealing with faulty positions of the toes. The three types of painful conditions may exist in the same foot, but more often one type predominates over the others.

Foot problems are more common among women than among men, and after women start wearing high heels, they tend to have more difficulty associated with the metatarsal arch and the toes than with the longitudinal arch. Men and children who present foot problems are prone to have those associated with longitudinal arch strain.

Pronation is an alignment fault in which weight is thrust toward the inner border of the foot. In those who wear low heels, such a fault places undue stress on the longitudinal arch structures. In women who wear high heels, the painful symptoms associated with this fault are often referred to the knee, or even the low back, rather than to the foot itself. This occurs because by raising the heel the bones of the foot are thrust into the structural relationship of a high longitudinal arch, and maintained there.

Examination of faulty and painful feet should include the following:

1. Check the alignment of the feet in standing with and without shoes.
2. Observe the manner of walking with and without shoes.
3. Test for muscle weakness or tightness of toe and foot muscles.
4. Check the shoes for over-all fit etc. (see p. 188), and observe the places of wear on the sole and heel. Faulty weight distribu-

tion in standing or walking is often revealed by excessive wear on certain parts of the shoe.
5. Check the over-all postural alignment for any evidence of superimposed strain on the feet such as occurs in cases of postural faults in which the body weight is borne too far forward over the balls of the feet.
6. Check regarding unfavorable occupational influences.

Treatment may be considered as of two types, corrective and palliative. Ideally, treatment should be corrective, but in view of the fact that many painful foot conditions occur in older people whose bony, ligamentous, and muscular structures cannot adjust to corrective measures, it is necessary to use measures designed to obtain relief with a minimum of correction.

The questions frequently are asked, "Should a person with weak feet wear arch supports or will he need to wear them the rest of his life if he starts wearing them?" "Should he be given foot exercises or are his feet already overworked?"

Except among individuals who have been bedridden or who do very little walking, it is safe to assume that the average person with a foot problem does not lack exercise. The activity or the type shoe that is worn, however, may hold the foot in such a position that muscles work at a disadvantage with the result that they suffer stretch-weakness and strain. There is no lack of use but there is diminished range of motion.

The foot muscles cannot be expected to fully compensate for or correct a condition in which there is faulty bony alignment and ligamentous relaxation. However, strong muscles will help preserve the alignment once it is corrected. Often a support is necessary until correction of alignment is satisfactory. The support should aim to relieve strain on the muscles. Normal use of the foot usually provides sufficient exercise for strengthening the muscles. However, stretching movements to relieve the tightness in muscles which maintain a persistent faulty alignment of the foot or toes may be indicated. Effective shoe corrections do much to bring about the gradual stretching of the tight muscle.

The list of exercises included may be considered primarily for use in cases of pronated feet or relaxed longitudinal arches. A few of these active movements once a day along with any necessary heat or massage of the tight muscles may be useful.

Recognition of the need for general postural correction is an important part of examination and treatment of faulty foot conditions.

Name: Date:

Corrective Foot Exercises

Lying on back:
1. Curl toes down and hold while pulling foot up and in.
2. Curl toes down and hold while pulling foot down and in.
3. With legs straight and together, try to touch soles of feet together.

Sitting in chair:
4. With (left) knee crossed over (right), move (left) foot in half circle, down, in, and up, then relax. (Do not turn foot outward.) Repeat with right foot.
5. With knees apart, place soles of feet together and hold while bringing knees together.
6. Place towel on floor. With feet parallel and about 6″ apart, grip towel with toes and pull inward with both feet, bunching towel between feet. Reach forward with toes (not out to side), grip towel again and repeat the movement.
7. With small half ball* under anterior arch of foot grip toes down over ball.

Standing:
8. With feet straight ahead, roll weight to outer borders of feet by pulling up under arches.

Walking:
9. Walk along a straight line on the floor, pointing toes straight ahead, and transferring weight from heel along outer border of foot to toes.

---

* Ball about $1\frac{1}{4}''$ to $1\frac{1}{2}''$ in diameter, cut in half.

Shoe Corrections

Since correction of faulty foot conditions is largely dependent on shoe alterations, brief descriptions of some of these are pertinent to this discussion. (Basic requirements for a shoe are discussed on p. 188, and shoe alterations are illustrated in fig. 131.)

Heel wedge is a small piece of leather made in the shape of half of the heel. It is usually applied between the (leather or rubber) heel lift and the heel proper. It is of a given thickness, usually $\frac{1}{16}''$ to $\frac{1}{8}''$, at the side and tapers off to nothing at the midline of the heel. An *inner wedge* is so placed that the thickness appears on the inner side of the heel and it serves to tilt the shoe slightly outward. In an *outer wedge* the thicker part is at the outer side of the heel and tends to tilt the shoe inward.

Sole wedge is made in the shape of a lengthwise one-half of the sole, and may be an inner or an outer wedge as in the case of the heel.

Thomas heel is a heel extended on the inner side for the purpose of medial longitudinal arch support. A *Reverse Thomas Heel* is extended on the outer side for correction of a supinated foot.

Longitudinal arch support is a support put inside the shoe under the medial longitudinal arch of the foot. It is usually made of sponge rubber and leather, although in some cases it is made of steel.

A *metatarsal pad* is a small sponge rubber pad made in an essentially triangular shape. It is placed back of the heads of the metatarsals and acts to reduce the hyperextension of the metatarsal-phalangeal joints of the second, third and fourth toes. To indicate the position of this support in *relation to the foot* and in *relation to the shoe* a metatarsal pad was inserted in a shoe and an x-ray of the foot was taken with the shoe on. The result is shown in fig. 132. (See also fig. 133.)

A *metatarsal bar* is a strip of leather extending across the back part of the sole of the shoe. It acts to lift the metatarsals just back of the heads as does the pad, but is more rigid and affects the position of all the toes rather than just the second, third and fourth.

Long counter is an extended counter which is added on the inner or outer side of the shoe. See fig. 131c. Fig. 134 shows the collapse of shoes in which there is no heel counter.

Faulty and Painful Conditions and Treatment Indications

PRONATION WITHOUT FLATNESS OF THE LONGITUDINAL ARCH

This type of fault is most often found among women who wear high heels. In weight-bearing there may be some symptoms of foot strain in

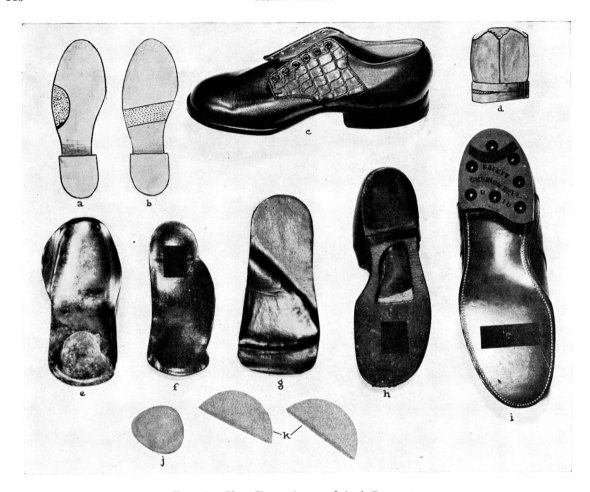

FIG. 131. Shoe Corrections and Arch Supports

a) Pigeon-toe patch; b) metatarsal bar; c) long inner counter (as indicated by the crease from the heel to the mid-section of the shoe); d) inner heel wedge; e) steel arch support for longitudinal and metatarsal arches; f) sponge rubber and leather support for support of longitudinal arch, and support of metatarsal arch at heads of 2nd and 3rd metatarsals; g) longitudinal arch support and metatarsal bar which supports all 5 metatarsals; h) sole of shoe cut out to show steel shank; i) modified Thomas Heel; j) small metatarsal pad; k) cork inserts to increase height of longitudinal arch support.

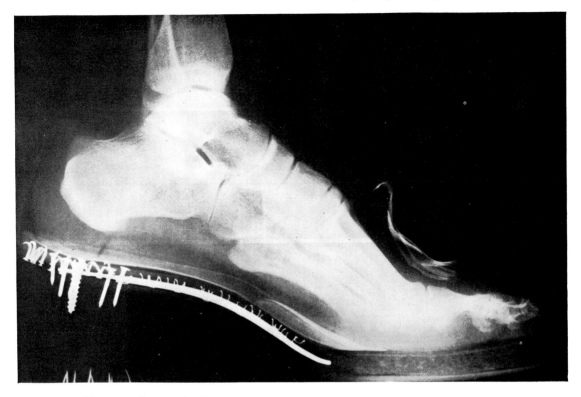

FIG. 132. X-ray of a Foot in a Shoe with the Subject in a Standing Position

The above illustration shows the proper relationship of a metatarsal pad to the foot and to the shoe. Observe that the thickness of the pad is posterior to the heads of the first four metatarsals. This illustration also shows how the steel shank supports the mid-section of the shoe and foot. The $\frac{1}{2}''$ platform sole reduces the relative height of the $2\frac{1}{4}''$ heel to the equivalent of a $1\frac{3}{4}''$ heel.

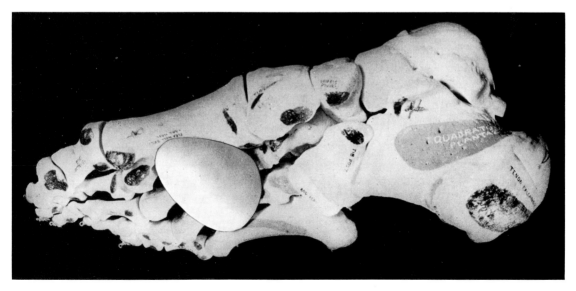

FIG. 133. A Metatarsal Pad Shown in Relation to the Metatarsal Bones

A metatarsal pad should be placed back of the heads of the metatarsals to avoid pressure at the joint surfaces.

the longitudinal arch structures and some evidence of undue compression laterally because of the limited range of eversion when in the position of plantar flexion as occurs in high heels. More often, however, the stress from the pronation fault causes strain medially at the knee. Because of the height of the heel the foot itself is subjected to more anterior arch strain than longitudinal arch strain.

Treatment consists of the use of an inner heel wedge. As a general principle, the patient should be discouraged from wearing a high heel if there are symptoms of foot or knee pain, but it may not be advisable for the patient to wear too low a heel. Furthermore, a high heel cannot be safely altered by use of a wedge without interfering with stability. On a heel of medium height, a $\frac{1}{16}''$ inner wedge is usually used while a $\frac{1}{8}''$ wedge is the usual adjustment on a low heel.

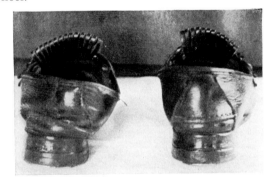

Fig. 134. Shoes Without Stiff Heel-Counter
The absence of a stiff counter in the heel allows the foot to deviate inward or outward. The shoe breaks down and any existing fault tends to become more pronounced.

PRONATION WITH FLATNESS OF THE LONGITUDINAL ARCH

This position of the foot is comparable to a position of dorsi-flexion and eversion. In weight-bearing the position of pronation with flatness of the longitudinal arch is usually accompanied by an outflaring of the forefoot. Excessive tension is exerted on the muscles and ligaments on the inner side of the foot which support the longitudinal arch. Undue compression is exerted on the outer side of the foot in the region of the

sinus tarsi where the astragalus and os ccisal articulate.

The tibialis posticus and abductor hallucis are usually weak, as also may be the toe extensor muscles and the flexor brevis digitorum. The peroneal muscles tend to be tight if pronation is marked.

Supportive treatment consists of using an inner heel wedge and a longitudinal arch support. When the heel has a wide base a wedge of $\frac{1}{8}''$ thickness is most often used. When the fault is severe, the patient should be discouraged from wearing a shoe without a heel. This type of fault is more often found among men or children than among women.

METATARSAL ARCH STRAIN

This type of strain is usually the result of wearing high heels, or of walking on hard surfaces in soft-soled shoes. It may also result from an unusual amount of jumping or hopping. An interesting and unusual example of the latter was observed in a child about ten years of age who had won a hop-scotch tournament. The foot on which she did most of her hopping had developed metatarsal strain and a callous on the ball of the foot.

The lumbricales, the adductor hallucis (transverse and oblique) and the flexor digiti quinti are most noticeably weak. When the patient is asked to flex the toes and "cup" the front part of the foot he is unable to do more than flex the end joints of the toes; there is no movement of cupping of the metatarsals.

Heat, massage, and stretching of the toe extensors is indicated if tightness exists. Supportive treatment consists of the use of a metatarsal pad or of a metatarsal bar. If there is a callus under the heads of the second, third, and fourth metatarsals usually a pad is indicated; if there is evidence of undue pressure as observed by calluses under the heads of all the metatarsals a bar is indicated.

OUTFLARE POSITION OF THE FEET

An outflare position may be the result of external rotation of the entire extremity from hip level, or tibial torsion in which the shaft of the tibia has developed a rotation, or may be a fault of the foot itself in which the forefoot flares out in relation to the posterior part of the foot.

The external rotation of the extremity may be seen in fig. 148. Such a position does not necessarily cause difficulty in standing but walking in an out-toed position tends to put strain on the longitudinal arch.

If tibial torsion is present as an established fault in an adult, no effort should be made to have the individual walk with the feet straight ahead because such "correction" of the foot position would result in a faulty alignment of the knees.

The outflare of the forefoot is the result of a breakdown of the longitudinal arch. In children measures which correct the arch position will help to correct the outflare. Wearing corrective shoes may be advisable because they typically have an inflare. In adults, however, if the fault is established, corrective shoes do not change the alignment of the foot but rather cause undue pressure on the foot. Usually it is necessary to have the patient wear shoes which have been made over a straight last or even an "out-flare last". The patient can tolerate some arch support and inner wedge alterations if these are indicated but the alignment of the shoe must necessarily conform to that of the foot to avoid pressure.

Toeing out in walking may result from tightness of the tendo-Achillis, in which case stretching of the plantar flexor muscles is indicated.

INFLARE POSITION OF THE FOOT

An inflare position of the feet may, like the outflare, be related to faults of position at various levels. The term *pigeon-toes* which refers to an in-toeing position may be considered as synonymous with inflare.

If the legs are internally rotated at the hips and there is no compensatory outward rotation at the lower leg or foot, the foot assumes an in-toeing position. Although muscle tightness in general is uncommon among children, it is not uncommon to find that the tensor fascia lata, which is an internal rotator, is tight in children who exhibit this fault. It is also interesting to note that children with this fault are inclined to sit on the floor in a position of internal rotation of the thighs, knock-knees and abduction of the lower legs so that one foot is on either side of the buttocks. The position may be termed reverse tailor-fashion.

Encouraging the child to assume a cross-legged position (tailor-fashion) tends to offset the effects of the other position.

Occasionally heat, massage, and stretching of the tensor are indicated.

The shoe correction used in cases of in-toeing associated with internal rotation of the extremity is a small, essentially semi-circular, patch placed on the outer side of the sole at about the base of the fifth metatarsal (see fig. 131a). To mark the area for the patch the shoe is held upside down and bent sharply at the sole in the manner it bends in walking. The patch extends about equally forward and backward from the apex of the bend. It is cut so that it is of a given thickness (either $\frac{1}{8}''$ or $\frac{3}{16}''$, depending on the size of the shoe) along the outer border. It tapers off to zero toward the front, center and back of the sole.

In-toeing associated with internal rotation of the extremity tends to be more marked in walking than in standing, and the shoe correction helps to change the walking rather than the standing pattern. However, the effect of changing the walking pattern in turn helps correct the standing position.

The patch, by its convex shape, pivots the foot outward as the sole of the shoe is brought in contact with the floor in the usual transfer of weight forward. Before marking the shoe for alteration, a leather patch may be taped to the sole of the shoe and tested for position by observing the child's walk.

When shoe alterations fail to bring about a correction of the in-toeing, a "twister" is used. (See fig. 135.) This consists of a strong elastic strap about 2″ wide which is attached to a belt around the pelvis. Fastened to the belt at the back, the strap extends diagonally across the buttocks, spirals around the thigh crossing diagonally in front, then spirals around the lower leg to attach to the outer sole of the shoe in front of the base of the 5th metatarsal.

An inflare position due to malalignment of

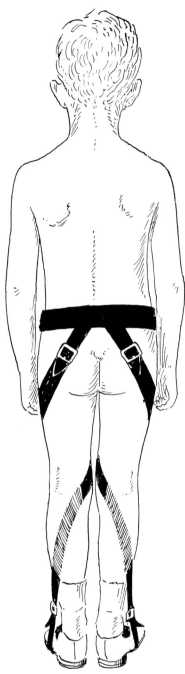

FIG. 135. Twister

The above figure shows a "twister" which is used to help correct in-toeing of the feet. (Whitman referred to this device as a Pigeon-toe Strap.)

Attached to a belt at center back, a wide band of non-elastic and strong elastic webbing spirals around the leg and is attached to the outer side of the sole of the shoe as illustrated. The shading represents the part of the band which is made of elastic.

To use the twister for correction of out-toeing the strap is attached to the belt in front, spirals around the leg, and is fastened to the inner side of the sole.

the forefoot in relation to the rest of the foot is similar to a mild club foot except that there is no supination of the heel or equinus. As a matter of fact, there may be pronation of the heel along with the forefoot inflare.

Inflare shoes may be comfortable but will not be corrective. The child should be fitted with shoes that have a straight last. A stiff inner counter extending from the base of the first metatarsal to the end of the great toe should be added to the shoe. The outer counter should be stiff from the heel to the cuboid.

SUPINATED FOOT

A supinated foot is a very uncommon postural fault (see fig. 50). It is essentially the reverse of a pronated foot and the shoe corrections are essentially the opposite of those applied to a pronated foot. An outer wedge on the heel, a reverse modified Thomas heel, and an outer sole wedge are usually indicated.

If knock-knee is associated with supination of the foot, shoe corrections as described above may increase the deformity of the knee. Careful consideration should be given to associated faults.

HALLUS VALGUS

A hallux valgus is a position of faulty alignment of the big toe in which the end of the toe deviates toward the midline of the foot, sometimes to the point of over-lapping the other toes. (See fig. 53.) The abductor hallucis muscle is stretched and weakened, and the adductor hallucis muscle is tight.

Such cases may require surgery if the fault cannot be corrected or pain alleviated by conservative means. However, in early stages it may be possible to affect considerable correction.

The patient should wear shoes which have a straight inner border, and should avoid the use of shoes with cut out toe space. A "toe-separator" which is a small piece of rubber that is inserted between the big toe and the second toe, aids considerably in holding the big toe in more normal alignment. As a purely palliative procedure for the relief of pain due to pressure, a "bunion-guard" is often useful.

HAMMER TOES

The position of hammer toes (as illustrated in fig. 54) is one in which the toes are hyperextended at the metatarsal-phalangeal joint and flexed at the interphalangeal joints. Usually there are calluses under the ball of the foot and corns on the toes as a result of pressure from the shoe.

Some massage and stretching may aid in correcting the faulty alignment of the toes in the early stage, and benefit may be obtained from a metatarsal bar. An inside metatarsal bar (as illustrated in fig. 131g) may be more effective, but an outside metatarsal bar (fig. 131b) is more comfortable.

CHAPTER IX

PAINFUL CONDITIONS OF THE UPPER BACK, NECK, ARM

The subject matter of this chapter deals with the problems of muscle imbalance or faulty posture in relation to painful conditions of the upper back, neck, and arm. Although the various conditions are described separately, it is not uncommon to find that they appear in combination. As the low back, pelvis, and legs are closely related in patterns of painful conditions, the upper back, neck, and arm are likewise closely related. The upper trunk is directly affected, too, by changes in alignment of the pelvis and low back, and it is often necessary to begin correction of faulty alignment of the upper trunk, where the painful symptoms exist, by support and postural correction of the abdomen and low back.

Upper Back

The problem in regard to upper back postural pain varies considerably from that of low back postural pain. In the low back, muscles are usually over-developed and frequently show adaptive shortening, and treatment consisting of heat, massage, and stretching of the contracted muscles is indicated. On the other hand, upper back muscles are usually weak and stretched. Treatment which relieves strain, as well as that which aids in the restoration of strength of these muscles, is indicated.

Middle and Lower Trapezius Strain

"Middle and Lower Trapezius strain" refers to the painful upper back condition resulting from a gradual and continuous tension on the middle and lower trapezius muscles. It is a rather prevalent condition, and one which is usually chronic. It seldom has an acute onset although the chronic symptoms may reach a point of severe pain.

The stretch-weakness of the muscles that precedes the condition of chronic muscle strain may result from an habitual position of forward shoulders or round upper back, or the combination of these two faults.

It may also occur as a result of the shoulders being pulled forward by overdevelopment and shortening of the anterior shoulder-girdle muscles. For some women, heavy breasts which are not adequately supported may also contribute to the faulty upper back and shoulder position.

Though the chief problem is one of undue tension on the posterior muscles, there is also a problem of undue compression on the anterior surfaces of the bodies of the dorsal vertebrae. Symptoms of muscle strain may occur in young adults, but symptoms of undue compression usually do not appear except in older people.

Symptoms associated with the muscle strain are at first those of soreness and fatigue progressing to a "burning" type pain along the course of the lower and middle trapezius.

In those individuals who exhibit no initial or adaptive shortness of the pectoral muscles, symptoms of pain are not constant. Recumbency or change of sitting posture may remove the element of continuous tension on the trapezius, and thus relieve the symptoms. Those individuals who have tightness in the pectoral muscles have continuous tension on the lower and middle trapezius. Change of position of the individual does not change the alignment of the part when such tightness exists. Pain, therefore, is relieved very little if at all by recumbency in cases of marked tightness.

When symptoms become acute an element of traction by the muscle on its bony attachments along the spine is added to the factor of muscle strain. Patients may complain of a sore spot, or palpation may elicit pain or acute tenderness in the region of the dorso-lumbar attachment of the lower trapezius.

Tests for length of the pectorals and other internal rotators and adductors should be done to determine the presence or absence of the tightness factor. If tightness is present, heat, massage, and gradual stretching of the tight muscles is indicated. There should be some effective relief in a short time if gentle treatment is given daily.

Whether tightness exists or not, a shoulder support is indicated. It is needed to aid in holding the shoulders back in a position that relieves tension on the trapezius. In the cases in which the weight of the breasts seems to be a factor in contributing to faulty position of the upper back, an uplift type of brassiere as shown in fig. 121 is indicated. If no tightness is present, some relief may be expected with the application of the support. If tightness of the muscles is present, relief of strain will be gradual, depending on the release of the muscle tightness.

For those cases (usually among older people) who have a fixed kyphosis position of the spine, little correction can be obtained. Some correction of the forward shoulders may be possible but the basic faults cannot be altered. A Taylor brace (fig. 123) may be used to give some relief from painful symptoms.

Heat and massage to the upper back over the painful area of muscle strain should be avoided. Such measures merely serve to further relax the already stretched muscles. After a support has been applied, and along with treatment to correct muscle tightness, exercises may be given to strengthen the lower and middle trapezius muscle. The exercise of pulling the elbows back against the wall with the arms up beside the head, and pulling the arms back against the wall in a diagonally overhead position are the two movements specific for strengthening this muscle. See fig. 138 A, B and C, and exercise sheet p. 115. The exercises shown in fig. 139 as contra-indicated for cases of coracoid pressure are also contra-indicated in cases of middle and lower trapezius strain.

Those cases in which there is a round upper back often develop symptoms in the posterior neck. As the dorsal spine bends into a kyphosis, the head is carried forward, and to preserve the erect position of the head, the cervical spine is necessarily hyperextended (see fig. 136). Symptoms associated with this fault are de-

scribed below under Pain Associated with Tightness of Posterior Neck Muscles.

Sports, such as baseball, may contribute to overdevelopment of the pectoral muscles. Occupations which require continuous work sitting at a desk contribute to the stretching of the trapezius muscles. A draftsman, for example, who sits on a high stool bent forward over his task, or a laboratory technician continuously bent over a microscope, is subjected to such a strain.

NECK

The muscle problems associated with pain in the posterior neck are essentially of two types, one associated with muscle tightness and the other with muscle strain. Symptoms and treatment indications differ according to the underlying fault. Both types are quite prevalent; the one associated with muscle tightness usually has a gradual onset of symptoms, while the one associated with muscle strain usually has an acute onset. The first is being labeled *Pain Associated with Tight Posterior Neck Muscles*, the second, *Upper Trapezius Strain*.

Pain Associated with Tightness of Posterior Neck Muscles

Symptoms of pain associated with tightness in the posterior muscles of the neck are most often found in patients who have a forward head and round upper back. As shown in fig. 136, the compensatory head position associated with a slumped, round upper back results in a position of hyperextension of the cervical spine.

The faulty mechanics associated with this condition consists chiefly of undue compression posteriorly on the articulating facets and posterior surfaces of the bodies of the vertebrae; stretch-weakness of anterior vertebral neck flexors; and tightness of neck extensors including the upper trapezius, splenius capitis, and cervical erector spinae. The apparent compression or impingement of the sub-occipital nerves, as they emerge through the fascial and muscular structure at the base of the skull, may account for the presence of "occipital headaches" that often occur along with the neck pain. The pa-

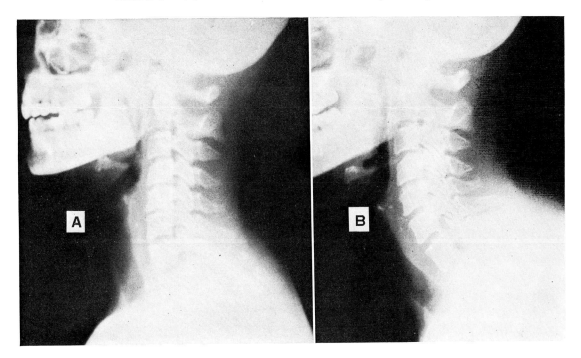

FIG. 136. X-rays of a Cervical Spine in Good and Faulty Positions

For the x-ray shown in fig. A the subject was sitting with the head and upper trunk in good alignment. The x-ray shown in fig. B is of the same subject sitting in a typically slumped position with a round upper back and forward head. As is illustrated the cervical spine assumes a position equivalent to that of hyperextension.

tient frequently complains of a feeling of "tension" in the back of the neck.

The extensor muscles are tight on palpation. Movements of the neck in all directions except hyperextension are limited to an extent that corresponds with the amount of tightness. Pain may be less in intensity when the patient is recumbent, but it tends to be present regardless of the position the patient assumes.

Treatment consists of the daily application of heat, massage and stretching. The massage should be gentle and relaxing at first progressing to deeper kneading. The stretching of the tight muscles must be very gradual, using both active and assisted movements. The patient should actively try to stretch the posterior neck muscles by efforts to flatten the cervical spine; i.e., pulling the chin down and in. This action compares with the effort to flatten the lumbar spine in cases of lordosis. Such exercises should be done in supine or sitting position, not in prone position. Any exercises which hyperextend the cervical spine are contra-indicated.

Because the faulty head position is generally compensatory to a dorsal kyphosis which in turn may result from postural deviations of the low back or pelvis, it is frequently necessary to begin treatment by correction of the associated faults. It is not uncommon to begin treatment for neck pain by the application of a good abdominal support which permits the patient to assume a better upper back and chest position.

Upper Trapezius Strain

The upper trapezius is that part of the trapezius muscle extending from the occiput to the acromion process of the scapula. A strain of this muscle results in pain, which is usually acute, in the postero-lateral region of the neck.

The stress that gives rise to this condition is often a combination of tension on, and contraction of, the muscle. Straining to reach for an object while holding the head tilted in the opposite direction may cause such an attack. The abduction of the arm requires action by the

trapezius in scapular fixation, and the sideways tilt of the head puts a tension on the muscle.

Over-all application of heat or massage tends to cause increased pain since the muscle is suffering strain. The part that is observed on palpation to be in a state of excessive contraction is the part treated. Since it is difficult to localize heat effectively to this small area massage alone is indicated. The movement is necessarily a kneading type of massage, gentle at first and more firm as the muscle tolerates the pressure. A treatment may require fifteen to twenty minutes of massage to effect relaxation. Pressure should be directed slightly upward to relieve the tension on the part of the muscle above. Downward stroking is at once irritating. It is advisable to apply an improvised collar if the irritation has been so marked that the localized treatment fails to bring relief. A simple collar can be made of cardboard, padded with cotton, and covered with gauze and fastened in front with adhesive; or a scarf wrapped around a piece of cardboard may be put around the neck and tied in place. Usually a day or two is as long as it will be necessary to wear such a support in the ordinary case of upper trapezius muscle strain.

ARM

Coracoid Pressure Syndrome

"Coracoid Pressure Syndrome"* refers to a condition of arm pain in which there is evidence of compression or irritation of the brachial plexus. It is associated with muscle imbalance and faulty postural alignment.

* This syndrome was recognized by the authors in 1942. It was first reported at a Joint Meeting of the Baltimore and Philadelphia Orthopedic Society, March 17, 1947, by E. David Weinberg, M.D., and subsequently referred to in an article by Dr. Irvin Stein entitled "Painful Conditions of the Shoulder Joint", The Physical Therapy Review, November–December, 1948, Volume 28, Number 6.

In 1945 an article was published by I. S. Wright in the American Heart Journal 29: 1–19 entitled "The Neurovascular Syndrome Produced by Hyperabduction of the Arms" in which a similar painful condition is described as occurring in association with the raised position of the arms.

At the level of the attachment of the pectoralis minor to the coracoid process of the scapula, the three cords of the plexus and the axillary artery and vein pass between these structures and the rib cage. (See fig. 137.) In normal alignment of the shoulder girdle there is no impingement on the nerves or blood vessels. Forward depression of the coracoid process as occurs in some types of faulty postural alignment, tends to narrow this space.

Forward depression of the shoulders with the coracoid process tilted down and forward may result from tightness of certain muscles pulling it into that position, or may be due to weakness of others allowing it to ride into that position. The painful arm conditions are more often found where the tightness factor predominates.

The muscle which acts to depress the coracoid process forward is chiefly the pectoralis minor. The upward pull of the rhomboids and levator scapulae posteriorly aid in the upward shift of the scapula that goes along with the forward depression. Tightness of the latissimus dorsi affects the position indirectly through its action to depress the head of the humerus. Pectoralis major tightness acts in a similar manner. In some instances, tightness of the biceps and coraco-brachialis which originate on the coracoid process along with the pectoralis minor seems to be a factor. Without attempting to differentiate each muscle tightness in testing, one may ascertain the presence or absence of tightness of this group of muscles by the arm-overhead extension test. (See figs. 97, 98 and 99.)

The muscle weakness which contributes chiefly to the faulty shoulder position is that of the lower trapezius. Stretch-weakness of this muscle allows the scapula to ride upward into a position favoring a forward depression. Such a position also favors an adaptive shortening of the pectoralis minor. (See fig. 99.)

Symptoms of pain may in some instances result from the pressure of a tight pectoralis minor, but when the alignment is very faulty and pain is constant, it suggests impingement between the bony prominence and the ribs.

In the acute stage, moderate or even slight pressure on the coracoid process usually elicits pain down the arm. Soreness is acute in that spot, and in the area described by the pectoralis minor muscle along the chest wall. The patient may be aware of symptoms of pain in the anterior chest area. In case of pain in the left arm and pectoral region, patients have often interpreted symptoms as a possible heart condition. Among women, pain on either side has frequently been interpreted as a breast lesion.

The pain down the arm may be generalized or may be predominately of lateral or medial cord distribution. There may be tingling, numbness, or weakness. The patient often complains of "loss of grip in the hand". Evidence of circulatory congestion with puffiness of the hand and engorgement of the blood vessels may be present. In case of marked disturbance the hand may be somewhat cyanotic in appearance.

The patient will complain of increased pain when wearing a heavy overcoat, or when trying to lift or carry a heavy weight with that arm.

Frequently, the area extending from the occiput to the acromion process, which corresponds to the upper trapezius muscle, is found to be sensitive and painful. This muscle is in a state of "protective spasm" in an effort to lift the weight of the shoulder girdle to relieve pressure on the plexus. It remains in a state of irritation until effective treatment is instituted.

Treatment in the acute stage consists first of applying a sling to support the weight of the arm, thus relieving the weight of the shoulder girdle on the plexus, and relieving the irritation in the upper trapezius. As soon as the acute pain has subsided heat and massage are applied to the upper trapezius and stretching of the tight pectoral muscles is instituted.

The patient is placed in a supine position with knees slightly flexed. The involved arm is placed in as much overhead extension as can be readily tolerated by the patient. Moderate heat (infra red, electric pad, or warm moist heat) is applied to the tight pectorals. Massage is applied which is at first gentle and relaxing,

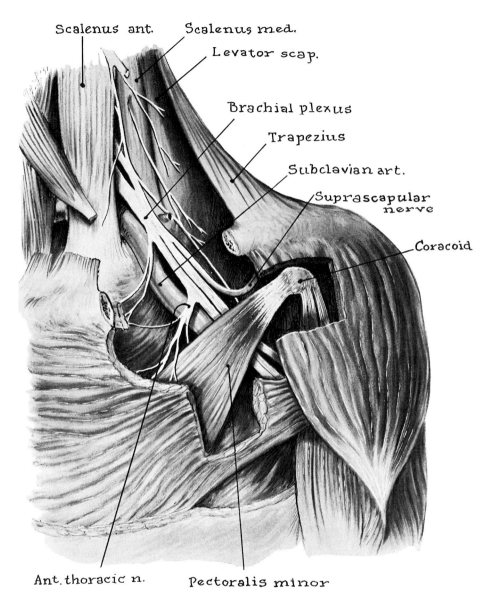

Scalenus ant.   Scalenus med.

Levator scap.

Brachial plexus

Trapezius

Subclavian art.

Suprascapular
nerve

Coracoid

Ant. thoracic n.   Pectoralis minor

FIG. 137. Relationship of the Brachial Plexus to the Coracoid Process and the Pectoralis Minor Muscle

and which, after a few treatments, progresses to being a gentle kneading and stretching massage. With one hand the therapist maintains an easy traction and gentle but steady pressure to stretch the patient's arm overhead, while massaging with the other. A figure-8 or other shoulder support (see fig. 122) is usually needed to maintain the correction of alignment and relieve strain on the lower trapezius muscle during the recovery period.

Though the associated muscle problems are usually the predominent factor, the faulty alignment in coracoid pressure syndrome may be due to the excessive pressure by the brassiere straps in women who have very large breasts. Correction in these cases is obtained by application of an uplift, strapless-type of brassiere. (See fig. 121.) A long brassiere (one which has a diaphragm band 2 or 3 inches wide) is reinforced with feather-bone stays which act to support the weight of the breasts from below. Straps may be left on the brassiere, but they should carry no weight if the support is effective.

After strain has been relieved by support and by stretching of tight opposing muscles, specific exercises are indicated for the middle and lower trapezius. (See fig. 138 and exercise sheet p. 115.)

If the over-all posture is faulty, general postural correction is indicated, along with specific correction of the shoulder girdle faults.

Contra-indicated are such exercises as the following:

Head and shoulder raising from a back-lying position because this movement tends to increase compression in the anterior shoulder region.

Shoulder adduction exercises which depress the head of the humerus and coracoid process forward. (See fig. 139.) This type of movement tends to exaggerate the existing fault.

Teres Syndrome

"Teres syndrome" refers to a condition of arm pain characterized by axillary and/or radial distribution of pain. Although pain of radial or axillary distribution may arise from posterior cord pressure at a higher level, it is the opinion of the authors that arm pain of this type in many cases arises from the level of the teres major and minor.

The axillary nerve emerges between the teres major and minor to supply the deltoid, while the radial nerve continues under the teres major and long head of the triceps to spiral around the humerus and supply the muscles which extend the elbow, wrist, and fingers.

In the cases showing either axillary or radial distribution of pain, the teres major which is an internal rotator is tight and holds the humerus in internal rotation; the teres minor which is an external rotator is taut by being placed on a tension as a result of the internal rotation.

The arm tends to hang at the side in a position of internal rotation, i.e., the palm of the hand faces more toward the back than toward the side of the body.

There is an element of tension on the posterior cord and axillary branch produced by the position of the arm (see fig. 36). There may also be an element of compression of the nerve trunk around the head of the humerus. Pain is usually more marked in active motion indicating an element of irritation to the axillary nerve by the teres muscles in movement. Internal or external rotation, whether done actively or passively, is painful; external rotation is limited. With the limitation of external rotation, abduction movements are also painful because the humerus does not rotate outward normally as it should during abduction. The pain is not unlike that encountered in cases of sub-deltoid bursitis.

A slight or moderate pressure over the triangle between the teres major and minor may elicit sharp pain radiating into the deltoid region. When there is pain of radial distribution, palpation over the long head of the triceps and elbow extension against resistance tends to be painful.

Treatment consists of applying heat and massage to the under arm and pectoral regions to stretch the internal rotators of the humerus. Stretching of the arm in overhead extension and in external rotation is done very gradually. In the stretching, an effort is made to have the

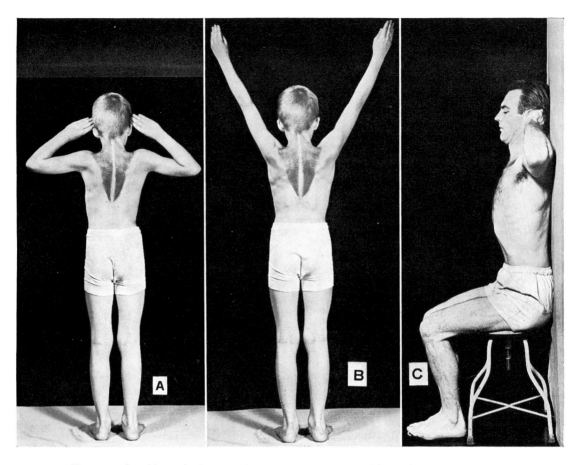

FIG. 138. Specific and Therapeutic Exercises for the Middle and Lower Trapezius

The trapezius muscle is illustrated by the markings on the skin in the above illustration.

Fig. A shows an exercise specific for the middle trapezius; fig. B an exercise specific for the lower trapezius. Fig. C shows a middle trapezius exercise being done while sitting with back to a wall. The combination of movements to correct low back and head position while doing the trapezius exercise makes this a therapeutic exercise for correction of the postural faults present.

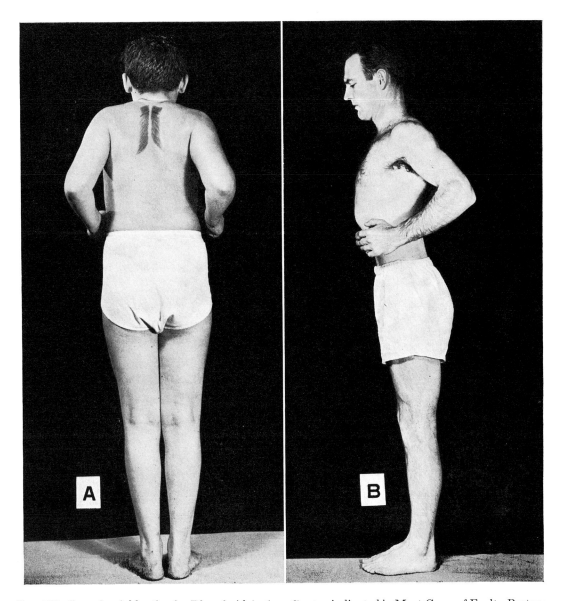

FIG. 139. Scapular Adduction by Rhomboid Action, Contra-indicated in Most Cases of Faulty Posture

The markings on the skin in fig. A indicate the position of the rhomboid muscles. The movement of scapular adduction with the arms in the position illustrated is brought about chiefly by the rhomboids. Fig. B shows the same movement from side view. The head tends to be thrust into a forward-head position and the shoulders are depressed forward in relation to the chest during this exercise.

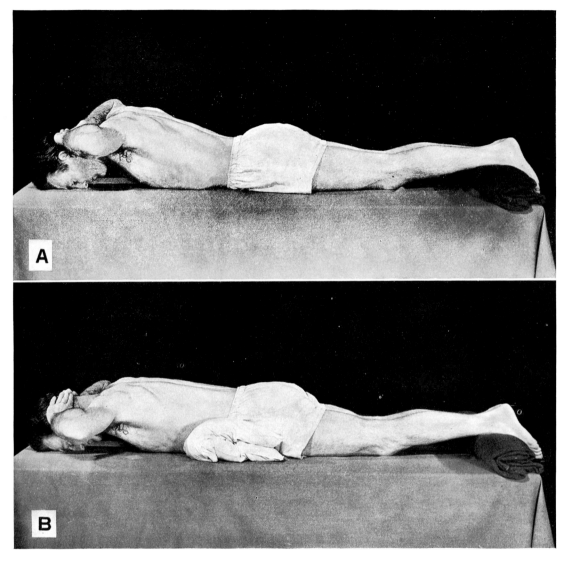

FIG. 140. Trapezius Exercise in Prone Position

Although the sitting position is preferable for doing the trapezius exercise, it is sometimes necessary to do the exercise from a prone position. The arching of the low back and the position of the head forward in relation to the upper back, as seen in fig. A, should be minimized as much as possible by placing a pillow under the abdomen as shown in fig. B and by not raising the elbows too high.

assistant hold the scapula back to effectively localize the stretching to the scapulo-humeral muscles rather than to the muscles which attach the scapula to the spine, namely the trapezius and the rhomboids. These latter muscles are often already stretched by the abducted position of the scapulae.

Cervical Nerve Root Pressure

Just as the sciatic pain caused by a protruded lumbar disc is basically a neurological problem, so also is the arm pain due to cervical nerve root pressure. It should be noted, however, that faulty posture of the cervical spine may act as a contributory factor in such cases when the onset is not associated with sudden trauma.

Hyperextension of the cervical spine as seen in a forward head position (see fig. 136) produces undue compression on the facets and posterior surfaces of the bodies of the cervical vertebrae. Conservative treatment may be adequate or it may be an adjunct to surgical measures.

Conservative treatment requires the application of a collar to relieve compression, before measures are instituted to correct any underlying faults in alignment or muscle balance. Such a collar should not hyperextend the cervical spine, but should support the weight of the head by transmitting this weight to the shoulder girdle. At the same time the collar exerts *slight* traction on the cervical spine by an upward lift.

Cervical Rib

A cervical rib is a congenital bony abnormality which may or may not give rise to symptoms of nerve irritation. The posture of the individual with a cervical rib often determines whether or not painful symptoms will occur.

A painful arm condition appearing in young or middle-aged adults is occasionally found to be

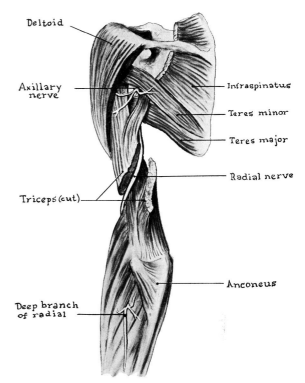

FIG. 141. Relationship of Axillary and Radial Nerves to the Teres Major and Minor, and Long Head of the Triceps

related to the presence of a cervical rib. In these cases the appearance of symptoms only after the person has reached adulthood may be explained by the fact that the posture of the individual has gradually become more faulty in alignment, thus causing the relationship of the rib and adjacent nerve trunks to change unfavorably.

The faulty alignment most likely to cause irritation is the type with forward head position. Care of a patient with painful symptoms due to cervical ribs requires postural correction of the upper back and neck. This treatment may relieve the symptoms completely and obviate surgical procedures.

PART IV

PREVENTION OF POSTURAL FAULTS

CHAPTER X

DEVELOPMENTAL FACTORS AND ENVIRONMENTAL INFLUENCES AFFECTING POSTURE

The preceding nine chapters have dealt with *Posture* and *Pain*, primarily in relation to the adult. This chapter aims to introduce a variety of concepts dealing with the development of postural habits in the growing individual and with a variety of influences which affect such development. No attempt is made to give the various concepts introduced either exhaustive or equal treatment. The authors hope that the material presented will be suggestive, and useful in a preventive sense; that it will create, through a recognition of factors involved in postural development, a more positive approach toward providing, within available limits, the best possible environment for good posture.

While it is important to observe and recognize marked or persistent postural deviations in the growing individual it is equally important to recognize that children are not expected to conform to an adult standard of alignment. This is true for a variety of reasons but primarily because the developing individual exhibits much greater mobility and flexibility than the adult.

Most postural deviations in the growing individual fall in the category of developmental deviations; when patterns become habitual they may result in postural faults. The developmental deviations are those which appear in many children at about the same age and which improve or disappear without any corrective treatment, sometimes even despite unfavorable environmental influences. However, in some individuals a developmental deviation is perpetuated by a faulty habit. Whether or not a deviation in a child is becoming a fault should be determined by repeated or continued observation, not by a single examination. If the condition remains static, or if the deviation increases, corrective measures are indicated. Any faults which are severe need treatment as soon as they are observed regardless of the age of the individual.

A young child is not very likely to have habitual faults and can be harmed by corrective measures that are not needed. Over-correction may lead to atypical faults more harmful and difficult to deal with than the ones which caused the original concern.

Some of the differences between child and adult are due to the fact that in the years between birth and maturity the structures of the body grow at varying rates, and in general grow rapidly at first and then at a gradually reduced rate. An example of this is the increase in size of the bones. Associated with increased over-all length of the skeleton is a change in the proportionate lengths of its various segments. This change in proportions occurs as first one part of the skeleton and then another has the most rapid rate of growth. The gradual tightening of ligaments and fascia and strengthening of muscles is a significant developmental factor. Its effect is to gradually limit the range of joint motion toward that typical of maturity. The increase in stability that results is advantageous because it decreases the danger of strain from handling heavy objects or from other strenuous activities. Normal joint range for adults should provide an effective balance between motion and stability. A joint which is either too limited in range or not sufficiently limited is vulnerable to strain.

The child's greater range of joint motion makes possible momentary and habitual deviations in his alignment which would be considered distortions in the adult. At the same time it seems to protect him to a considerable degree against getting fixed postural faults.

Since the primary functions of muscles are to move the body and to contribute to its support the degree of muscular strength needed has a direct relation to the size and weight of the body and its various parts. Thus, though a child's musculature may be normally strong at any given age, his strength must continue to develop as his height and weight increase. In general, then, muscle strength in children and adults is not equal but the relative strength of the various muscles is comparable.

Beginning in infancy there is a persistent imbalance between the strength of the front and back muscles of the trunk and neck. The greater strength of the posterior muscles permits the child to raise his head and trunk backward long before he can raise either forward without assistance. Although the abdominal and neck flexor muscles never do match the strength of their opponents they are much stronger relatively in the adult than in the child. Thus in this regard an individual should not be expected to conform to the adult standard until he approaches maturity.

Good postural development is to a considerable degree dependent upon good structural and functional development of the body which is in turn highly dependent upon adequate nutrition. The influence of nutrition upon the proper structural development of skeletal and muscular tissues is of particular significance. Rickets, for example, which is often responsible for severe skeletal deformities in children, is known to be a deficiency disease.

After growth is completed, poor nutrition is less likely to cause structural faults which directly affect posture. At this stage deficiencies are more likely to interfere with physiological function and to be represented posturally in positions of fatigue. The body uses food not only for growth, but also for fuel, transforming it into heat and energy. If the fuel is insufficient there is a loss of energy output and in the body it is seen as fatigue and a decrease in general physiological efficiency. Nutritional deficiencies in the adult are most likely to occur when unusual physiological demands are made upon the individual over a period of time.

The relationship between sound development and adequate nutrition is recognized, as is that between nutrition and maintenance of the energy level and of good physiological function; it may be said that nutrition is of primary importance in all aspects of health and development and in like manner it is important in the development and maintenance of good posture.

There are physical defects, diseases, and disabilities which have associated postural problems; these conditions can be roughly divided into three groups insofar as attention to posture is of importance in their treatment.

The first group consists largely of physical defects in which the postural aspects are more potential than actual in the initial stages, and become a problem only if the defect cannot be completely corrected by medical or surgical means. These defects may be visual, auditory, skeletal such as club foot or dislocation of the hip, neuromuscular such as brachial plexus injury, or muscular such as wry neck.

The second group includes conditions which are in themselves potentially disabling, but in which continuing attention to posture from the early stages can minimize the disabling effects. In arthritis deformans of the spine, for example, if the body can be kept in a good functional alignment during the time that fusion of the spine is taking place, the individual may have little obvious deformity and only moderate disability when the fusion is complete. If the postural aspect is disregarded, the trunk is usually in marked flexion when fusion of the spine is complete. This is a position of severe deformity and of associated severe disability.

In the third group are conditions in which a degree of permanent disability exists as a result of injury or disease, but in which added postural strain can greatly increase the disability. An amputation of the lower extremity, for example, throws an unavoidable extra burden on the remaining weight-bearing structures. A postural alignment which minimizes, as much as possible, the mechanical strains of position and motion does much to keep these structures from breaking down. (See figs. 142 and 143.)

A consideration of normal and abnormal variations in the posture of children can be discussed both from the standpoint of over-all posture, and from the standpoint of the deviations of the various segments. Variations in over-all posture of children of approximately the same age are illustrated in figs. 144 and 145. Deviations of the various segments of the body are discussed in the following paragraphs.

A small child's foot is normally flat when he begins to stand and walk. The bones are in a formative stage and the arch structure is incomplete. The arch develops gradually along with the development of the bones, and with the strengthening of muscles and ligaments. By the age of six or seven one may expect good arch formation. Footprints taken at regular intervals help to gauge the amount of change that has occurred in the arch. These can be taken with a pedigraph, or if this is not available, the sole of the foot can be painted with vaseline and a footprint made on paper. As the arch increases in height, less of the sole of the foot in the area of the arch will be seen in the footprint.

Flat longitudinal arches may persist as a fixed fault or they may recur because of foot strain at any age. Improper shoes or a habit of standing and walking with the feet in an out-flare position may cause such strain. If a child's foot is very flat, is pronated, and flares out in a manner that allows the body weight to be borne constantly on the inner side of the foot, it may be necessary to use a slight correction such as inner heel-wedge or small longitudinal pad in the shoe quite soon after the child begins to stand and walk. In most cases, however, it is advisable to institute corrective measures only after a period of observation. There are individuals who fail to develop a longitudinal arch and have what is termed a static flat foot. Usually, however, the alignment of the foot is not faulty in regard to pronation or outflare, and there are no symptoms of foot strain. The corrective measures usually indicated for flat arches are not indicated in such cases.

A degree of knock-knee is common in children, and is usually first observed when the child begins to stand. The height and build of the child must be taken into consideration when judging whether the deviation is a fault, but in general it may be said that a fault exists if the ankles are more than two inches apart when the knees are touching. (See fig. 146.) As a child grows taller a two inch separation of his feet represents the normally smaller deviation at the knee expected in an older child. Knock-knee should be showing definite improvement before, and be non-existent by, the age of six or seven.

In some cases, knock-kneed children may stand with one knee (often the right) slightly flexed and the other slightly hyperextended so that the knees overlap in order to keep the feet together. Knock-knees may persist; in adults this fault is more prevalent among women than among men.

Records of the change in the degree of knock-knee can be kept by drawing an outline of the legs on paper while the child is lying or standing with his knees touching each other. Mild to moderate knock-knee conditions are usually treated by shoe corrections, while bracing or even surgery may be required for the more severe. (See fig. 130.)

Bow-legs is an alignment fault in which there is separation of the knees when the feet are together. It may be a postural or a structural fault. Postural bowing is a deviation associated with knee hyperextension. (See figs. 41 and 42.) As the posterior ligaments tighten and hyperextension decreases, this type of fault tends to become less pronounced. If it persists as a postural habit the child should be given instruction in order to correct the alignment faults. This fault is less easy to correct as the individual approaches maturity, although some degree of correction may be obtained in young adults who are very flexible.

Postural bow-legs may be compensatory for knock-knees. If a knock-kneed child stands with his legs thrust back into hyperextension, the resultant postural bowing of the legs will let him bring his feet together without having his knees overlap. In this position the knock-knee fault may be obscured, but it will become obvious if the legs are brought into a neutral position of knee extension. (See fig. 147.)

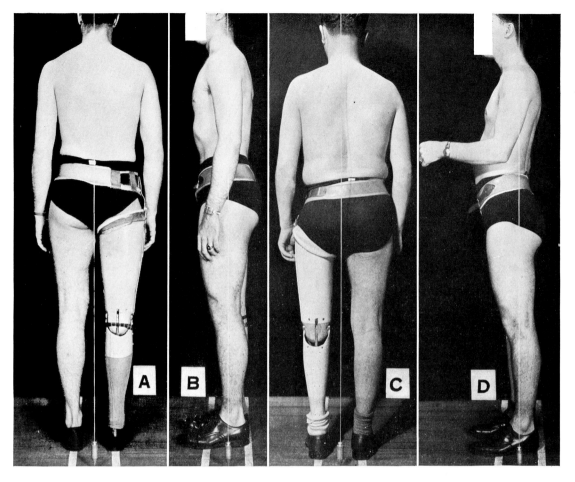

FIG. 142. Good and Faulty Position in Amputees

The subject shown in figs. A and B has good postural alignment which should hold to a minimum the extra stresses of weight-bearing associated with lower extremity amputation.

In figs. C and D the subjects have alignment faults which impose undue weight-bearing stresses in addition to those related to the amputation. It is most essential that an amputee be capable of good alignment before he is measured for a prosthesis. If a prosthesis has been fitted to conform to a faulty postural alignment the person usually cannot correct his alignment while wearing it even though a remedial program to correct the underlying muscle imbalance and faulty habits of position is undertaken.

Balancing the strength of the hip abductors through exercise and correcting any muscle tightness which exists before the prosthesis is applied helps to prevent such an alignment fault.

In fig. D the subject deviates forward above the hips. He has a severe lordosis and clockwise rotation of the pelvis and trunk. These faults combine to exert added stress on the low back region.

(Reproduced from Physical Therapy for Lower Extremity Amputees, War Department Technical Manual TM8-293, June 1946.)

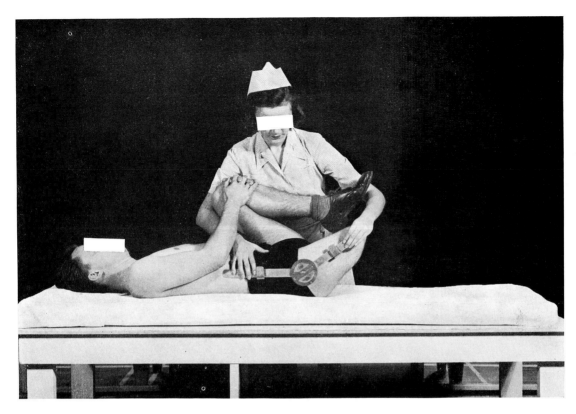

FIG. 143. Test for Hip Flexor Tightness

This figure shows the same subject as is seen in fig. 142D. The test for hip flexor tightness reveals a severe limitation of hip extension on the right. When the subject stands in his prosthesis the pelvis must be flexed on the thigh to the same degree that the thigh is flexed on the pelvis in this picture. Unless the hip flexion contractures are released it is impossible for a subject to assume a good standing position The subject pictured in A and B of fig. 142 showed good muscle balance when tested for muscle length and strength.

(Reproduced from Physical Therapy for Lower Extremity Amputees, War Department Technical Manual TM8-293, June 1946.)

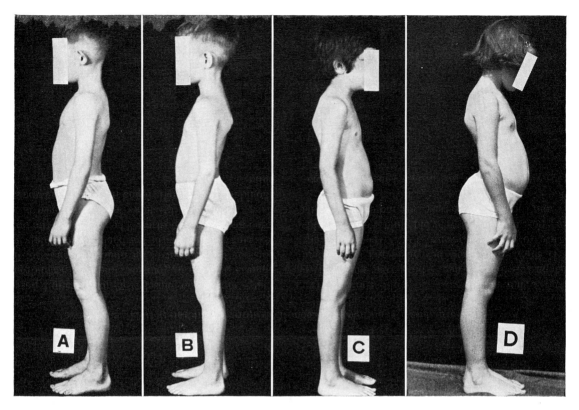

Fig. 144. Normal and Abnormal Variations in Posture of Children (6 to 8 years of age)

Fig. A shows a 7 year old child with unusually good posture for his age.

Fig. B shows an 8 year old boy with what may be considered average posture. The slight prominence of the shoulder blades seems to be typical of this age. The posture of the 6½ year old child as seen in fig. C may be considered somewhat faulty. Such a child needs observation and guidance for good postural development. Fig. D shows an 8 year old child with very faulty posture. Treatment consisting of the use of some form of corset for back and abdominal support, and therapeutic postural exercise are needed in such a case.

The contour of the abdomen and the increased forward curve of the low back illustrated in fig. B is characteristic of children of this age.

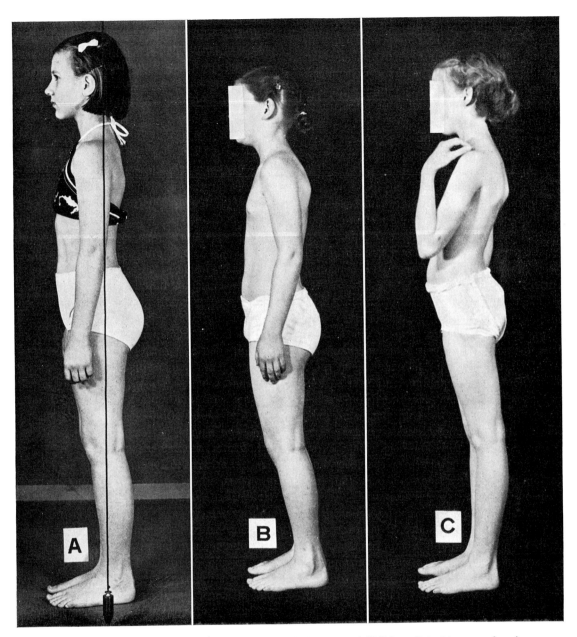

FIG. 145. Normal and Abnormal Variations in Posture of Children (9 to 11 years of age)

Fig. A shows a 10½ year old child who has very good posture for her age. The 9 year old child in fig. B shows what may be considered an average posture for this age group. Fig. C shows a very faulty posture in an 11 year old child. Postural guidance and therapeutic exercises are indicated for this child.

Observe that good posture at this age approximates much more closely the normal adult posture than is the case in younger children. In children of this age the contour of the abdomen tends to show less curve than does the low back in individuals with good and average posture. The contour of the upper back, also, typically shows less prominence of the shoulder blades than is found in the average younger child.

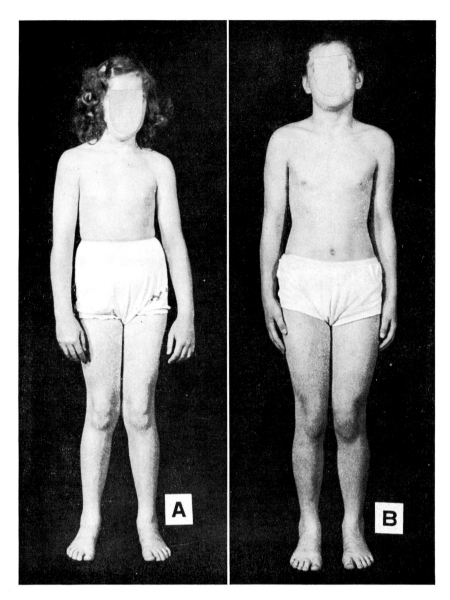

FIG. 146. Knock-knee, Severe and Mild

Fig. A shows a degree of knock-knee which may be considered a fault in a child of any age. The inner edges of the heels measured 5 inches apart. The knees show no signs of rotation. In a child of this age (8½ years) shoe corrections would not be adequate to bring about a correction. (See p. 142 regarding treatment.)

Fig. B shows a mild degree of knock-knee in a 9 year old girl. If this deviation has persisted from early childhood it may be tending toward a fixed fault. However, it is mild enough not to be a cause for concern. The internal rotation of the knees, however, is of a sufficient degree to warrant attention. Shoe corrections in the form of inner wedges on the heels, and postural exercises are indicated.

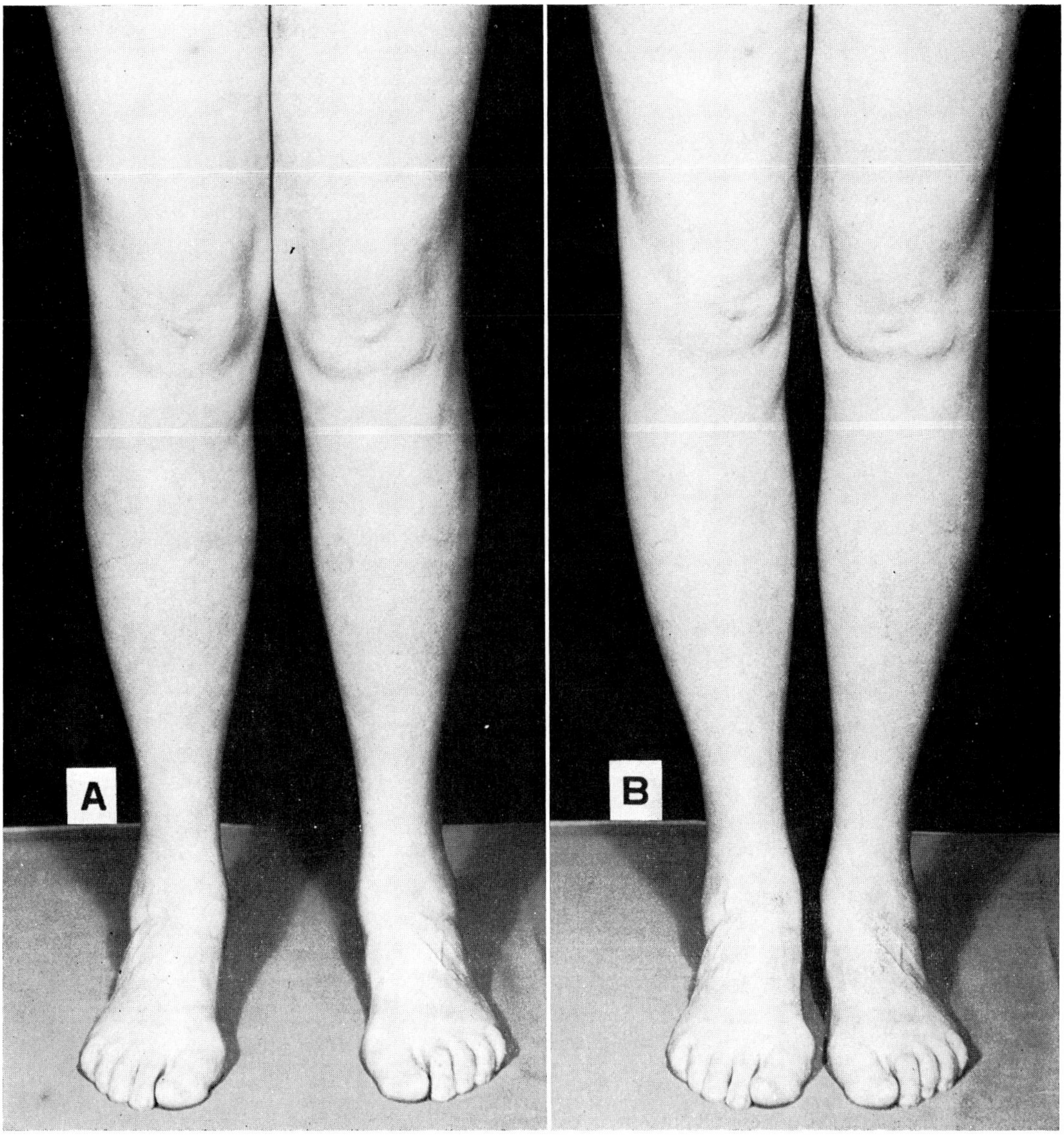

FIG. 147. Hyperextension Compensatory for Knock-knees

Fig. A shows the position of knock-knees which the subject exhibits when the knees are in good antero-posterior alignment.

Fig. B shows that by hyperextending her knees the subject is able to produce enough postural bowing to accommodate for the $4\frac{1}{2}$ inch separation of her feet in fig. A.

See figs. 41 and 42 for the extent of postural bowing which can be produced by hyperextension in an individual who has no knock-knee condition.

Children are often embarrassed by the appearance of knock-knees, and it is not uncommon for them to make this compensation habitually if the knock-knee condition is allowed to persist.

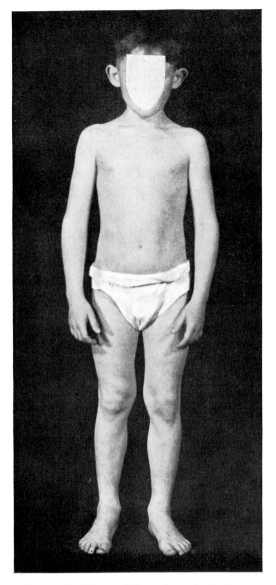

FIG. 148. External Rotation of the Legs

The external rotation of the legs as seen in this subject is the result of outward rotation at the hip joint. In other respects the alignment of the legs and feet is good.

Postural bowing usually disappears when an individual is recumbent, while structural bowing does not. Structural bowing requires early anti-rachitic treatment, or in later stages may require surgery.

Drawings to record the change in structural bow-legs can be made while the child is in a back-lying position with his feet together. Since postural bowing shows up only in standing, the drawing of this for record must be made in standing. It can be done by placing the paper on a wall behind the standing child.

Inward rotation of the femur, seen as a turning inward of the patella, is the most common alignment fault of the knees and may occur at any age. It frequently occurs in combination with other faults such as pronation of the feet, hyperextension of the knees, postural bow-legs, and less often with knock-knees. (See fig. 146 B.) When it is associated with postural bowlegs it usually disappears immediately when the legs are brought forward out of hyperextension. (See fig. 41.) Its permanent improvement depends upon the correction of the faulty habit of hyperextension. When associated with pronation and knock-knee the same shoe correction which helps one usually helps the others also.

Children may stand in a position of external rotation of the feet and knees. (See fig. 148.) Such a position is more typical of boys than of girls. It may or may not have serious effects, although persistence of such a pattern in walking as well as in standing may put undue strain on the longitudinal arches.

Hyperextension is a fairly common fault, usually associated with lack of firm ligamentous support. It tends to disappear as the ligaments tighten, but if it persists as a postural habit an effort should be made to correct it by postural training.

It is characteristic of small children to have a protruding abdomen. (See fig. 144.) For the most part, the contour of the abdominal wall changes gradually but there is a noticeable change about the age of ten or twelve when the waist line becomes relatively smaller, and the abdomen no longer protrudes.

Posture of the back varies somewhat with the age of the child. A small child may stand bent slightly forward at the hips (see fig. 149), and with feet apart for better balance. Children of early school age appear to have a typical deviation of the upper back in which the shoulder blades are quite prominent (see fig. 150). Beginning about the age of nine there seems to be a tendency for increased forward curve or lordosis of the low back. The deviations should tend to become less pronounced as the child grows older.

At an early age handedness patterns related to posture begin to become apparent. The slight deviation of the spine to the side opposite the higher hip makes an appearance early. There tends to be a compensatory low shoulder on the side of the higher hip. In most cases the low shoulder is a less significant factor. Usually shoulder correction tends to follow correction of lateral pelvic tilt, but the reverse does not occur. No attempt should be made to raise the shoulder into position by constant muscular effort.

The ability of individuals to touch the toes with the finger-tips while sitting with legs extended shows interesting variations according to age. Fig. 151 shows a series of drawings which indicate what is apparently normal accomplishment in this movement at different ages.*

The activities in which an individual engages may have favorable or adverse influence on posture. The nature of the activities, the time expended in them, and whether the effect of habitual movements is reinforced or counteracted by habitual positions determine to a great extent the postural effect.

The activities of an individual must be considered as a whole in gauging their postural effect. Concentration on one type of activity provides a high potential for muscle imbalance.

* Based on a study "Normal Flexibility According to Age Groups" by H. O. and F. P. Kendall, with a Foreword by George E. Bennett, M.D., reported in The Journal of Bone and Joint Surgery, Volume 30-A, Number 3, July, 1948, pp. 690–694.

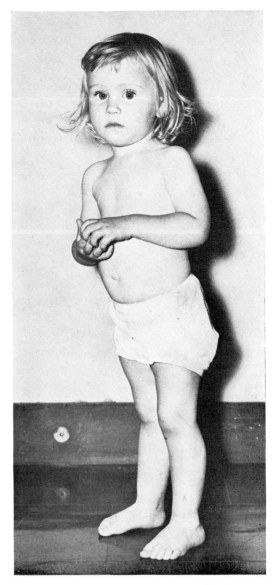

FIG. 149. Posture of Small Child

The flexed hips and wide stance of this $1\frac{1}{2}$ year old child suggest the uncertain balance associated with this age. Although it is not very evident in the picture, the subject had at this time a mild degree of knock-knee. (This deviation gradually decreased without any corrective measures so that at the present age of six, this child's legs are in good alignment.)

The development of the longitudinal arch in this subject is very good for a child of her age.

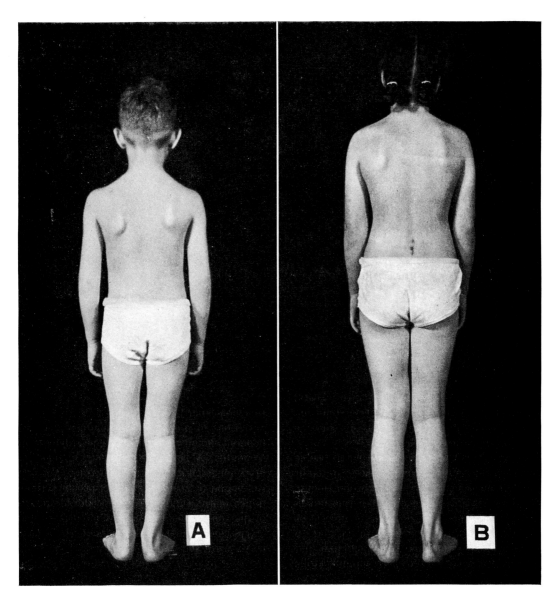

Fig. 150. Deviations of the Scapula

The degree of scapular prominence seen in fig. A is rather typical of children of this age (8 years). It need not be a matter of concern at this age even though the scapulae are relatively farther apart than in good adult posture. (For a side view of this subject see fig. 144B.)

The subject in fig. B is a 9 year old girl who is rather mature for her age. The forward position of the shoulders is typical of that assumed by many young girls at the time of beginning development of the breasts.

When such a postural habit becomes more marked and persists for a considerable period it may result in a fixed postural fault.

Although the scapulae are abducted, they do not appear as prominent as in the younger child shown in fig. A.

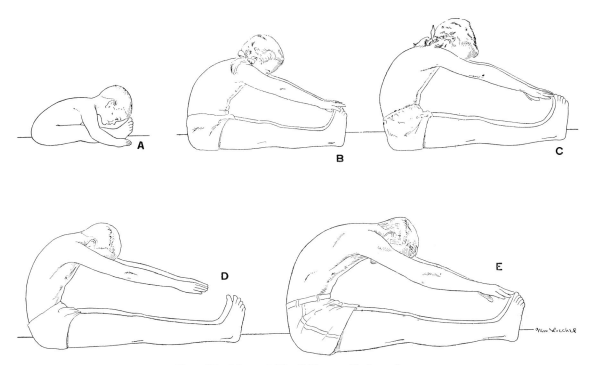

FIG. 151. Normal Flexibility at Various Ages

The ability to touch the toes with the finger tips may be considered normal for young children and adults. However, between the ages of 11 and 15 many individuals who show no signs of muscle or joint tightness are unable to complete this movement. The reason seems to be that the proportionate length of the trunk and lower extremities is different in individuals of this age group from that in people of younger and older age groups.

The five drawings in the figure are representative of the majority of individuals in each of the following age groups: Fig. A, 1 to 3 years; fig. B, 4 to 7 years; fig. C, 8 to 10 years; fig. D, 11 to 14 years; and fig E, 15 years and over.

The change from the apparently extreme flexibility of the youngest child to the apparently limited flexibility of the child in fig. D occurs gradually over the period of years as the legs become proportionately longer in relation to the trunk. For children, standards of performance which involve forward bending should take into consideration the normal variations in the ability to complete the range of this movement.

A combination of activities might have almost as unfavorable an effect if each of them involved the same kind of movement or position. For example, a typist who engages in sedentary activities such as piano playing during her leisure time has no real change in type of activity from the postural standpoint.

Activities which cause lateral deviations in the alignment may or may not cause fixed postural faults. Sometimes, as is shown in figs. 152 and 153, the deviations to the left and right tend to counteract each other. However, the tendency to assume positions which consistently cause a deviation to the same side may result in a fixed lateral curve.

Some deviations of alignment have no obvious relation to the activities of the individual, but are constant enough to be habitual faults. (See fig. 154.)

If changes of activity are to be compensatory they must give variety in position and movement. For anyone who has to sit long hours at a desk whether in school or at work, shifts of position or simple extension movements are usually possible and desirable. A sitting position keeps the hips, the knees, and usually the back in flexion. Relaxing against the back of the seat is a small but useful change from sitting with the trunk held forward as for writing at a desk. A true change of position would involve full extension of the body as in standing up or lying down.

The principle that activities should be varied for the sake of good posture is subject to sensible limitations in its application. It is not logical to assume that an individual's primary consideration in choosing his activities will be postural. However, he may be able to eliminate or minimize unfavorable postural influences intrinsic to the activities he engages in if he is aware of postural implications and makes any indicated adjustments whenever they are practical.

Although no recreational activities should be considered as having a positive therapeutic value in correcting postural faults, some may be considered as better balanced activities than others. Of these, dance movements which involve normal movements of the body are potentially the most valuable for preserving symmetry and muscle balance. The dancer should avoid extreme positions and should cultivate the ability to perform movements toward one side as easily as toward the other. Without these precautions dancing may lead to considerable distortion of alignment and to muscle imbalance. A fault sometimes seen in adults as a result of several years of acrobatic dancing at an early age is a flattening or reversal of the normal backward curve of the spine in the upper back. (See fig. 155.) It results from repeated hyperextension movements of the spine through an extreme range of motion persisted in during the period of growth when the bones are still in the formative stage. Individuals who begin dancing at a later age when the spinal curves are less susceptible to distortion rarely show this particular fault.

Some other activities which are rather neutral in their effect on posture are games or sports in which walking or running predominates. Sports activities which exert a rather definite influence toward muscle imbalance are the predominantly one-sided games, such as those involving the use of a racket.

The play activities of young children usually are varied enough so that no problem of muscle imbalance or habitual alignment fault is present. However, when a child becomes old enough to engage in competitive athletics he may reach a point where further development of his skill through intensive practice requires a sacrifice of some degree of good muscle balance and good skeletal alignment. Although seemingly unimportant at the time, the faults acquired may progress until a painful condition results.

Specific exercises may be needed to maintain range of joint motion and to strengthen the muscles whose opponents are being overdeveloped by the activity. These exercises must be specific for their purpose and therapeutic for the body as a whole.

Vocational activity is a more influential factor in the posture of the average adult than is his recreational activity. The repeated movements involved in a specialized occupation are the equivalent of repeated exercises, and thus may be responsible for overdevelopment of certain muscle groups. If the effect of poor position reinforces that of repeated activity the muscle imbalance is greatly increased.

There are a number of environmental factors which influence the development and maintenance of good posture. These environmental influences should be made as favorable to good posture as is practical; when no major adjustment is possible, small adjustments will often contribute considerably. The following discussion takes into account such factors as chairs, beds, and shoes because they illustrate environmental influences on posture in the sitting, lying, and standing positions. After a child starts school, the amount of time he spends in the sitting position increases considerably and the school seat is an important environmental factor.

The chair and desk should both be carefully adjusted to fit the child. The child should be able to sit with both feet flat on the floor with knees bent to about a right angle. If the chair is too high or too low either there is lack of support for the feet, or the hips and the knees are bent into too much flexion. The seat of the chair should be deep enough from front to back to support the thighs adequately but the depth should not interfere with the bending of the knees. The back of the chair should provide support for the child's back. It should also incline backward a few degrees so that the child can relax against the back of the chair. (See illustration of sitting postures, fig. 156.)

The top of the desk should be at about the level of his elbows when he is sitting in a good position, and may be slightly inclined. The desk should be close enough so that the child can rest his arms on it without having to lean too far forward or sit forward on the seat of the chair.

Generally speaking, the type and size of his chair is important to anyone who spends many hours in a sitting position. Whenever possible a chair should be selected which gives a maximum of comfort and support.

Not all chairs are conducive to good sitting position. So-called posture chairs which support the back only in the lumbar region tend to cause an increase in the lumbar curve and are often undesirable.

While it is advisable that the back of a chair be inclined slightly backward, it is not good to have too great an angle of backward tilt. Sitting for long periods of time in a swivel chair which tilts back may contribute to a very faulty position of the upper back and head. (See fig. 157.)

Automobile seats which are too low or which have been tilted backward somewhat for the comfort of the passengers may be unsatisfactory for the driver. Much of the pain and fatigue in the neck and shoulder region which are frequently associated with long periods of driving can be traced to the necessity for holding the head in a forward or tilted position. A firm wedge-shaped pillow (with wider part at the top) can be used to decrease the inclination of the back of the seat behind the driver.

The qualifications for height and proximity of the school desk apply to almost any work surface for a sedentary worker. Whenever it is practical tools and equipment should be placed where they may be reached without undue stretch or torsion.

The light provided for any activity should be of adequate intensity for the purpose and located so that it falls correctly on the work space. It should be free from glare, bright reflections, or unnecessary shadows.

The firmness of a mattress is an important factor in the consideration of posture in the lying position. A good sleeping position involves having the various parts of the body in about the same horizontal plane. Either sagging springs or too soft an inner-spring mattress may permit poor body alignment. The importance of a firm bed is demonstrated most dramatically in the cases of certain people who have experienced postural back pain; some have found that pain has been decreased or eliminated by changing from a sagging to a firm level bed. Others who have been accustomed to sleeping on a firm mattress have found that acute pain may be brought on by sleeping on a soft or sagging bed.

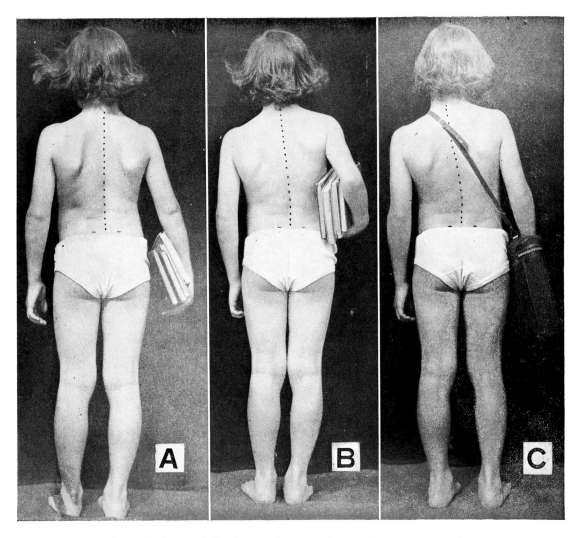

FIG. 152. Postural Deviations Associated with Common Activities

The above figure and the following one show an 8 year old girl in a number of positions representative of situations that are part of her every-day experience. In each case she was asked to assume the position that felt most natural and comfortable in the given situation. The common factor in the above is that each involves an asymmetrical position of the body.

The figures above show deviations of the spine associated with three common ways of carrying school books. The degree of deviation in a picture of a child can be only an indication of the general trend because the degree of deviation varies almost momentarily.

These pictures do not show the most marked deviations seen in this child, nor do they show the effects of fatigue from having maintained the position for any length of time.

Although fig. A appears to be the least faulty, it is not safe to assume that this position is preferred because this way of carrying books can displace the trunk sideways over the pelvis to a marked degree.

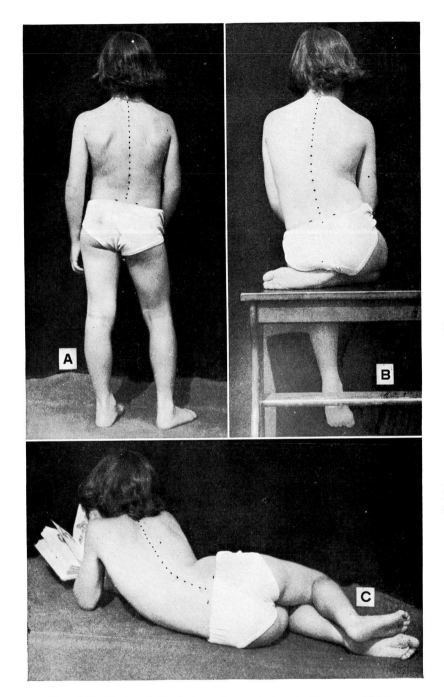

FIG. 153. Postural Deviations Associated with Common Habits

For fig. A above the child was asked to stand with her weight on one foot.

Deviations such as those illustrated are a natural result of ordinary activities and are not a cause for concern if the spine deviates almost as often to one side as to the other, and as long as no single pattern of deviation becomes habitual.

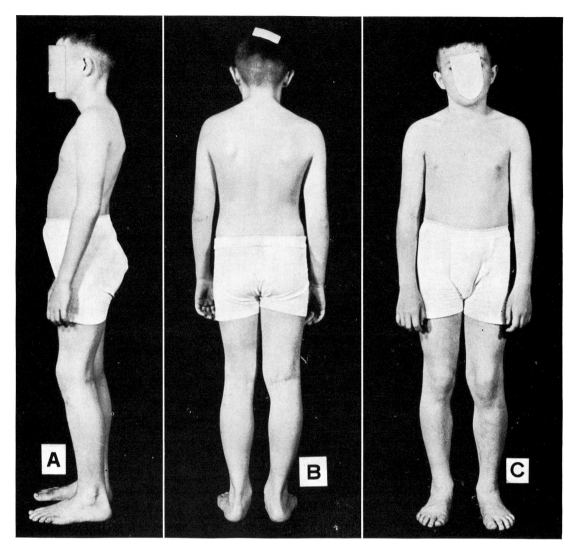

FIG. 154. Knee Flexion as a Postural Habit

This nine year old boy has a fairly typical posture for his age except for an habitual flexion of the left knee which is seen in each of the three views. Such a habit may eventually result in an inability to extend the knee completely. However, an even more immediate consideration is the fact that the fault in alignment of the knee joint has resulted in compensatory deviations of alignment in other parts of the body. The high right hip and low right shoulder in this child show a greater degree of deviation than would be expected at his age even though this is the basic pattern accompanying his right-handedness.

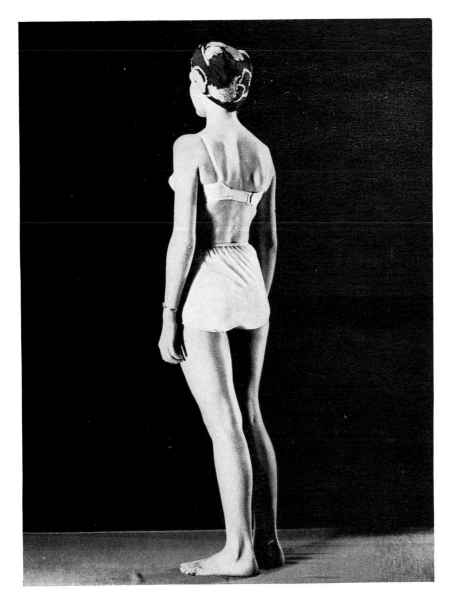

FIG. 155. Dorsal Lordosis in Dancer

This illustration shows a reversal of the normal posterior curve in the dorsal spine. As in this subject, this slight abnormality appears to be associated with repeated hyperextension movements as done in acrobatic dancing. This fault has been seen in numerous individuals who have had several years of acrobatic dancing starting at an early age. (The depression that is present in the dorsal area does not show up to best advantage in this illustration, but the oblique view was the only one in which it could be demonstrated.)

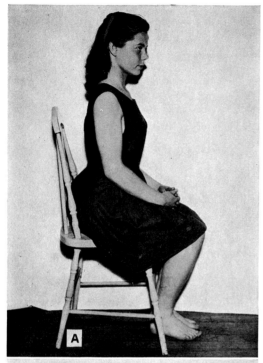

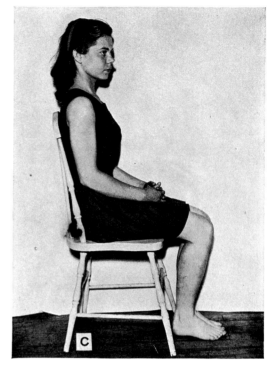

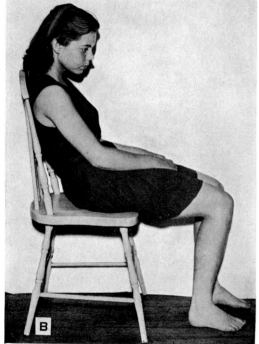

FIG. 156. Good and Faulty Sitting Positions

In fig. A the subject is "sitting up so straight" that the low back is in a lordosis. Such a position can be held only with effort. This is sometimes mistakenly considered a correct sitting position. A chair which supports the back only in the lumbar region is liable to cause such a position.

The position in fig. B results in lack of support for the low back and a very faulty position of both upper back and head.

The position in fig. C is good in regard to both alignment and ease.

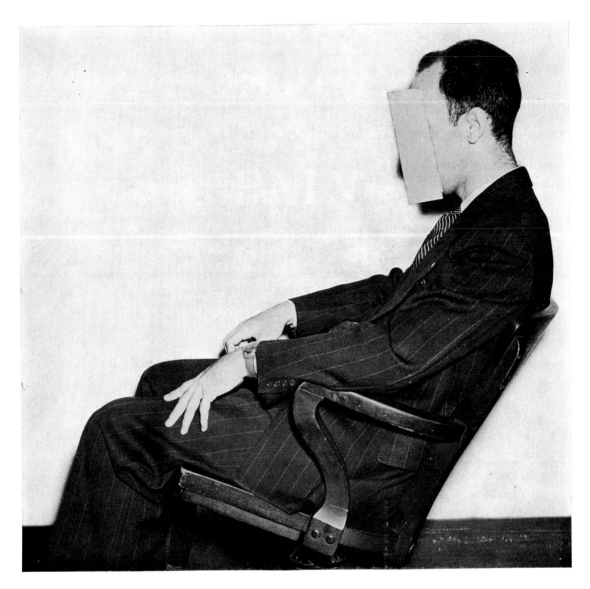

FIG. 157. Faulty Position of Head and Shoulders in Sitting

This figure illustrates the faulty alignment of the neck and upper back which results from sitting tilted back in a swivel chair.

For some individuals, particularly those who have fixed structural faults of alignment such as exaggerated curves of the spine, a softer mattress may be necessary for sleeping comfort because the mattress will give more support and comfort if it conforms to the curves than if it "bridges" them.

An infant should have a bed with a firm mattress. It may be somewhat softer than the mattress used by an adult because the weight of the infant does not cause the mattress to sag. The infant should sleep without a pillow.

When sleeping on his back or abdomen, an adult might be comfortable without a pillow, but in a side-lying position he probably would not be comfortable. Use of too high a pillow or more than one pillow may contribute to faulty head and shoulder positions. However, a person who is used to sleeping with his head high should not change abruptly to using a low pillow or none at all. This is especially true if the person has a fixed postural fault of forward head and round upper back. A gradual decrease in pillow height may be indicated but treatment to correct the faulty head position may need to accompany the change of position.

A discussion of posture is not complete without some reference to the principles of good body mechanics as applied to lifting and carrying heavy objects. Figs. 158 and 159 illustrate and describe some of the basic principles.

The protection and support given by shoes are important considerations in regard to the postural alignment in standing. Various factors predispose toward faulty alignment and foot strain, and create the need for adequate shoe support. The flat, unyielding floors and sidewalks of our environment, the use of heels which decrease the stability of the foot, and prolonged periods of standing as required in some occupations, are some of the contributing causes.

In the following paragraphs a number of factors relating to the size, shape, and construction of a shoe are discussed.

LENGTH

Over-all length should be adequate for comfort and normal function.

Length from the heel to the ball: Feet vary in arch and toe length, some having a longer arch and shorter toes while others have a shorter arch and longer toes. No special type of shoe is suited to all individuals, and one must find a shoe that fits in respect to arch length as well as over-all length.

WIDTH

A shoe that is too narrow cramps the foot; one that is too wide fails to give proper support or may cause blisters by rubbing against the foot.

Width of the heel "cup": The shoe should fit snugly around the heel of the foot. It is often a problem to find a shoe with a heel cup narrow enough in proportion to the rest of the shoe.

Width of the shank: The shank is the narrow part of the sole under the instep. The shank should not be too wide, but should permit the contour of the leather upper part of the shoe to be molded around the contour of the arch of the foot. If the shank is too wide the arch of the foot does not have the support given by the shoe counter.

Toe width: This needs to allow for good toe position and to permit action of the toes in walking. The toe-box or (toe counter) helps to give space to this part of the foot and keeps the pressure of the shoe off the toes.

SHAPE OF THE SHOE

A normal foot should be able to assume a normal position in a properly fitted shoe. Any distortion in shape that tends to pull the foot out of good alignment is not desirable. It is a fairly common fault that shoes "flare-in" too much. This design is based on the assumption that the long arch is relieved of strain because it is raised by an inward twist of the forefoot. The foot of a growing child may conform to the abnormal shape if such shoes are worn for a period of years. Because an adult's foot is not as flexible as a child's and is not easily forced out of its usual alignment, a shoe with an inflare is likely to cause excessive pressure on the toes.

HEEL COUNTER

A *heel counter* is a reinforcement of stiff material inserted between the outer and inner layers of leather which form the back of a shoe. It serves two purposes; to provide lateral support for the foot, and to help preserve the shape of the shoe. As the height of the heel increases, the lateral stability of the foot decreases and the counter becomes especially important for balance.

When the leather surrounding the heel is not reinforced it will usually collapse after a short period of wear and shift laterally in whatever direction the wearer habitually thrusts his weight. When this has happened the feet can no longer be held in a good alignment by such shoes. (See fig. 134.)

Shoes which have a cut-out back and depend upon a strap to hold the heel in place offer even less stability than do shoes with enclosed heels and no counter. The shoe itself does not show as much deterioration with wear because the strap merely shifts sideward with the heel, and there is no heel leather to break down. In flat-heeled shoes the effect on the wearer may be minimal, but the lack of lateral support in a higher heel cannot persist indefinitely without some ill effects. The effects may be felt more at the knee than in the foot itself.

STRENGTH OF THE SHANK

A good *shank* is of prime importance both for the durability of the shoe itself and for the well-being of the person who wears it. When a shoe has a heel of any height the part of the shoe under the instep is off the floor. The shank must then be an arch-like support which bridges the space between the heel and the ball of the foot. If the shank is not made of a strong enough material it will sag under a normal load when the shoe is worn. Such a sag permits a downward shift of the arch of the foot, and tends to drive the toe and heel of the shoe apart. The extreme of this type of deterioration in a flat heeled shoe is sometimes seen in the rounded, rocker-bottom shape that results, the shank being lower than the tip of the toe or back of the heel.

A strip of steel reinforcing the shank provides the strength required to preserve the shoe as well as to protect the wearer from foot strain. (See fig. 132.) Both low and high heeled shoes require a strong shank. Fortunately most high-heeled shoes are made with good shanks. Low heeled shoes often are not. A prospective buyer can judge the shank of a shoe to some extent by placing the shoe on a firm surface and pressing downward on the shank with his fingers. If such moderate pressure makes it bend downward, it it safe to assume it will break down under the weight of the body.

In heel-less shoes such as sandals or tennis shoes the firmness of the shank is of little importance for a person with no foot problems. Because the whole foot is supported by the floor or ground, support from the shoe is not a major consideration, unless the foot is being subjected to unusual strain from activity (as in athletics) or strain from prolonged standing.

SOLE AND HEEL OF THE SHOE

Thickness and *flexibility* are the two important factors in judging the *sole* of a shoe. For prolonged standing especially on hard floors of wood, tile, or concrete, a thick sole of leather or rubber is desirable. It has some resiliency and is able to cushion the foot against the effects of the hard surface.

For people who are required to do a great deal of walking, a firm sole is desirable. The repeated movement of transferring weight across the ball of the foot in walking is a source of continuous strain. A firm sole which restricts an excessive bend at the junction of the toes with the ball of the foot guards against unnecessary strain. The sole should not be so stiff, however, that there is a restriction of normal movement in walking.

When a child is learning to walk, his shoes should have no heel and a sole flat and firm enough to give stability. The sole should be fairly flexible, however, to allow the proper development of his arch through walking.

The height of the heel is important in relation to strain of the arches of the foot. Wearing a heel changes the distribution of body weight,

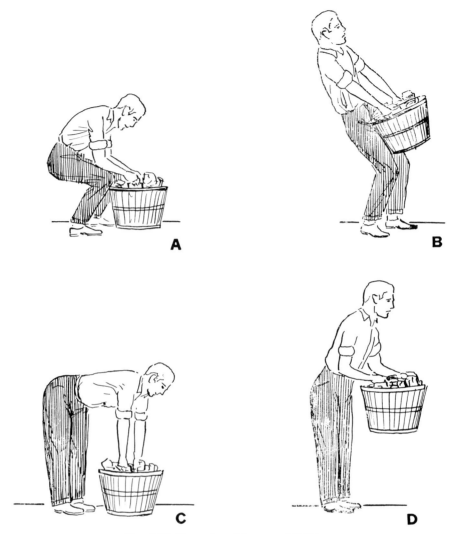

Fig. 158. Correct and Incorrect Lifting

Care should be taken in lifting a heavy object. When possible, one should stoop to pick it up as shown in fig. A, and carry it by bracing it against the thighs as shown in fig. B. Fig. A also shows the subject bracing his elbows on his thighs, giving support to the arms in order to initiate the lifting. One should avoid lifting and carrying heavy objects in the manner illustrated in figs. C and D because of the excessive strain imposed on the low back and hips.

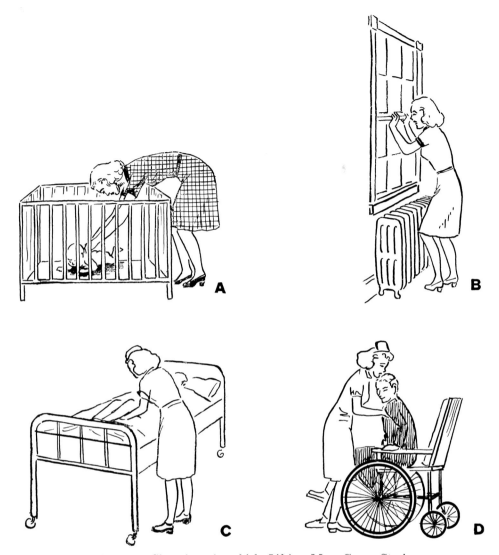

FIG. 159. Situations in which Lifting May Cause Strain

Each of the above illustrations shows a common situation in which the general rules about stooping to lift heavy objects cannot be applied. In each there is an element of hazard because it requires a degree of forward-bending at the hips that subjects the lifter to possible back strain.

However, the fundamental principles of good body mechanics should be applied in so far as possible. As shown in figs. A and B, the feet should be separated for balance, and, if possible, one foot should be placed slightly ahead of the other. The knees should be bent slightly. In leaning over, particularly as shown in figs. C and D, the back should not be allowed to arch but should be flattened by "tucking the hips under." Obviously, the person who has tightness of the low back muscles cannot assume this position of the back and hips and he is, therefore, more susceptible to strain from lifting than is the person with normal flexibility.

shifting it forward. The proportion of weight borne on the ball of the foot increases directly with the height of the heel. Continuous wearing of high heels eventually results in anterior foot strain.

The effects of a fairly high heel can be offset, but only to a limited degree, by the use of metatarsal pads and by wearing shoes which help to counteract the tendency of the foot to slide too far toward the toe of the shoe. An Oxford-type shoe which laces at the instep or a pump with a high-cut (and preferably elasticized) *vamp* help to restrain the foot from sliding forward by providing an evenly-distributed and uniform pressure if the shoe fits well.

When the foot is allowed to slip forward in the shoe, the toes are wedged into too small a space and subjected to considerable deforming pressure.

From the standpoint of normal growth and development as well as normal function, it is advisable that a person use a well constructed shoe with a low heel. However, there are individuals, especially women with a painful condition of the longitudinal arch, who are benefited by wearing shoes with heels of medium height. The higher heel mechanically increases the height of the longitudinal arch, and a flexible foot which is subject to longitudinal arch strain may be relieved of symptoms by using a heel about $1\frac{1}{2}$ inches high.

POSTURE INSTRUCTION

Good posture is not an end in itself but a part of general well-being. Ideally, posture instruction and training should become a part of general experience rather than be a separate discipline. To the extent that parents and teachers are cognizant of good postural habits and able to recognize the influences and habits which tend toward development of good or faulty posture— to that extent they will be more able to contribute to this aspect of well-being in the daily life of the growing individual. Nevertheless, posture instruction and training should not be neglected in a good program of health education; certainly direct and competent attention should be paid to observable faults. When instruction is given as such it should be simple and accurate; while it must not be neglected, neither should it be over-emphasized. It should be given in such a manner as to capture the interest and utilize the cooperation of the child.

While correction of postural defects requires the use of special therapeutic measures, the prevention of faults depends largely on teaching the fundamentals of good alignment. The following chart describes posture in relation to the various segments of the body in terms of both good and faulty alignment. An attempt has been made to present the material in a manner that makes it useful for the layman.

A CHART OF

POSTURAL INSTRUCTIONS

Part	Good Posture	Faulty Posture
Foot	In standing, the longitudinal arch has the shape of a half dome. Barefoot or in shoes without heels, the feet toe out slightly. In shoes with heels the feet are parallel. In walking with or without heels, the feet are parallel and the weight is transferred from the heel along the outer border to the ball of the foot. In running the feet are parallel or toe-in slightly. The weight is on the balls of the feet and toes because the heels do not come in contact with the ground.	Low longitudinal arch or flat foot. Low metatarsal arch, usually indicated by calluses under the ball of the foot. Weight borne on the inner side of the foot. (Pronation.) "Ankle rolls in". Weight borne on the outer border of the foot. (Supination.) "Ankle rolls out". Toeing out while walking, or while standing in shoes with heels. "Outflared" or "slue-footed". Toeing in while walking or standing. "Pigeon-toed".
Toes	Toes should be straight, that is, neither curled downward nor bent upward. They should extend forward in line with the foot and not be squeezed together or overlap.	Toes bend up at the first joint and down at middle and end joints so that the weight rests on the tips of the toes. (Hammer toes.) This fault is often associated with wearing shoes that are too short. Big toe slants inward toward the mid-line of the foot. (Hallux valgus.) "Bunion". This fault is often associated with wearing shoes that are too narrow and pointed at the toes.
Knees and Legs	Legs are straight up and down. Knee caps face straight ahead when feet are in good position. Looking at the knees from the side, the knees are straight, i.e., neither bent forward nor "locked" backward.	Knees touch when feet are apart. (Knock-knee.) Knees are apart when feet touch. (Bow-legs.) Knee curves slightly backward. (Hyperextended knee.) "Back-knee". Knee bends slightly forward, that is, it is not as straight as it should be. (Flexed knee.) Knee-caps face slightly toward each other. (Internally rotated femurs.) Knee-caps face slightly outward. (Externally rotated femurs.)
Hips, Pelvis and Spine	In general the body weight is borne evenly on both feet and the hips are level. One side is not more prominent than the other as seen from front or back, nor is one hip more forward or backward than the other as seen from the side. (Since a tendency toward a slightly low right shoulder and slightly high right hip is frequently found in right-handed people, and vice versa for left-handed, such deviations should not be considered abnormal.) The front of the pelvis and the thighs are in a straight line. The hips do not look prominent in back but slope slightly downward.	One hip is higher than the other. (Lateral pelvic tilt.) Sometimes it is not really much higher but appears so because a sideways sway of the body has made it more prominent. (Tailors and dressmakers often notice a lateral tilt because the hemline of skirts or length of trousers must be adjusted to the difference.) The hips are rotated so that one is farther forward than the other. (Clockwise or counter-clockwise rotation.) The low back arches forward too much. (Lordosis.) Also called "sway-back". Goes along with a pelvis that tilts forward too

Part	Good Posture	Faulty Posture
Hips, Pelvis and Spine—*Cont.*	The spine has four natural curves. In the neck and lower back the curve is forward, in the upper back and lowest part of the spine (sacral region) it is backward. The sacral curve is a fixed curve while the other three are flexible. The spine does not curve to the left or the right side. (A slight deviation to the left in right-handed individuals and to the right in left-handed individuals should not be considered abnormal, however.)	much. The front of the thigh forms an angle with the pelvis when this tilt is present. The normal forward curve in the low back has straightened out. The pelvis tips backward and there is a slightly backward slant to the line of the pelvis in relation to the front of the hips. (Flat back.) Increased backward curve in the upper back. (Kyphosis or round upper back.) Increased forward curve in neck. Almost always accompanied by round upper back and seen as a forward head. Lateral curve of the spine in either or both directions. (Scoliosis.)
Abdomen	In young children up to about the age of 10 the abdomen normally protrudes somewhat. In older children and adults it should be flat.	Entire abdomen protrudes. Lower part of the abdomen protrudes while the upper part is pulled in.
Chest	A good position of the chest is one in which it is slightly up and slightly forward (while the back remains in good alignment). The chest appears to be in a position about half way between that of a full inspiration and a forced expiration.	Depressed, or "hollow-chest" position. Lifted and held up too high, brought about by arching the back. Ribs more prominent on one side than on the other. Lower ribs flaring out or protruding.
Arms and Shoulders	Arms hang relaxed at the sides with palms of the hands facing toward the body. Elbows are slightly bent, so forearms hang slightly forward. Shoulders are level and neither one is more forward or backward than the other when seen from the side. Shoulder blades lie flat against the rib cage. They are neither too close together nor too wide apart. In adults a separation of about 4″ is average.	Holding the arms stiffly in any position forward, backward, or out from the body. Arms turned so that palms of hands face backward. One shoulder higher than the other. Both shoulders hiked-up. One or both shoulders drooping forward or sloping. Both shoulders rotated either clockwise or counter-clockwise. Shoulder blades pulled back too hard. Shoulder blades too far apart. Shoulder blades too prominent, standing out from the rib cage. "Winged scapulae".
Head	Head is held erect in a position of good balance.	Chin up too far. Head protruding forward. Head tilted or rotated to one side.

INDEX